8/06

Mediterranean Women Stay Slim, Too

Eating to Be

Sexy,

Fit, and

Fabulous!

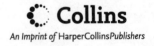 **Collins**

An Imprint of HarperCollins*Publishers*

Mediterranean Women Stay Slim, Too

Chef Melissa Kelly

with Eve Adamson

Produced by Amaranth

This book contains advice and information relating to health care. It is not intended to replace medical advice and should be used to supplement rather than replace regular care by your doctor. It is recommended that you seek your physician's advice before embarking on any medical program or treatment. All efforts have been made to assure the accuracy of the information contained in this book as of the date of publication. The publisher, the book producer, and the author disclaim liability for any medical outcomes that may occur as a result of applying the methods suggested in this book.

MEDITERRANEAN WOMEN STAY SLIM, TOO. Text copyright © 2006 by Amaranth Illuminare. Recipes copyright © 2006 by Melissa Kelly. All rights reserved. Printed in the United States of America. No part of this book may be used or reproduced in any manner whatsoever without written permission except in the case of brief quotations embodied in critical articles and reviews. For information address HarperCollins Publishers, 10 East 53rd Street, New York, NY 10022.

HarperCollins books may be purchased for educational, business, or sales promotional use. For information please write: Special Markets Department, HarperCollins Publishers, 10 East 53rd Street, New York, NY 10022.

FIRST EDITION

Designed by Jaime Putorti

Map of the Mediterranean by Wendy Frost

Printed on acid-free paper

Library of Congress Cataloging-in-Publication Data has been requested.

ISBN-10: 0-06-085421-9
ISBN-13: 978-0-06-085421-8

06 07 08 09 10 WBC/RRD 10 9 8 7 6 5 4 3 2 1

To women everywhere seeking a healthier, more beautiful, more conscious way of living: mothers, daughters, sisters, and grandmothers, links in the chain of healthy vibrant women throughout the United States, the Mediterranean, and across the globe. And to the men behind us who encourage and love us: our partners, our fathers, our sons, our brothers, and our grandfathers. Salut!

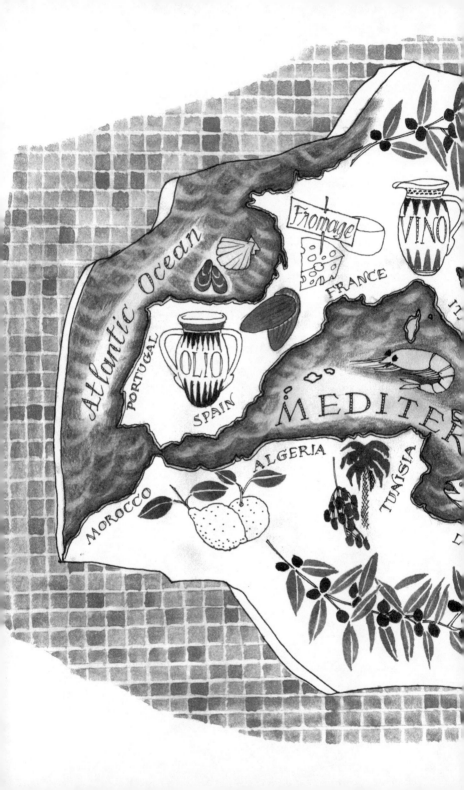

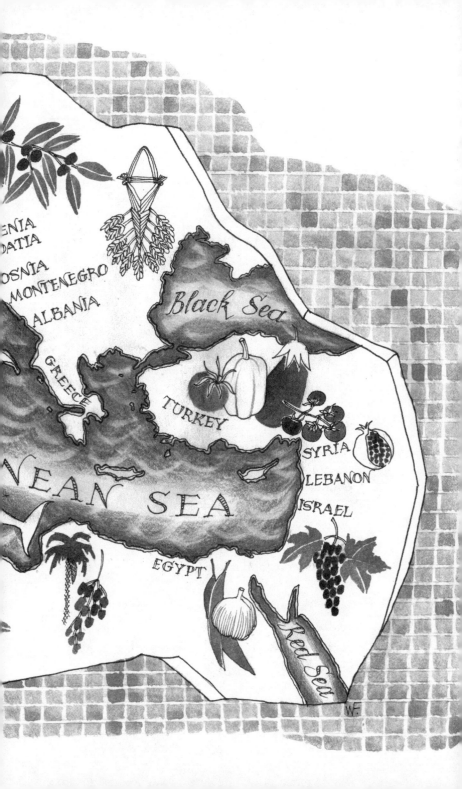

Contents

Alpha

You don't have to speak Greek to know that *alpha* symbolizes beginnings. The first letter of the Greek alphabet, alpha implies potential and all that lies ahead. To me, alpha also represents the beginning of a journey, a transformation, and an adventure. Are you feeling adventurous? Are you ready for a change in your life? Do you want to come along with me?

Where would you like to go, and how would you like to look and feel when you get there? Are you thinking southern France, where chic French women spend hours browsing through the local open-air market to find the perfect piece of fruit? How do they find the time, and how do they acquire such good taste? How do they prepare food so that it is just perfectly *délicieux*?

Maybe Italy is more your style, with its passion, gusto, and boisterous meals that last for hours *con la tua famiglia*. Or perhaps you are enchanted by the thought of Barcelona, where you can sip sherry and nibble on tapas and gaze upon the magnificent architecture with your animated Spanish friends. *Esto está eccelente!* Or maybe you imagine yourself as a Greek goddess with gorgeous curves and flowing robes, strolling through the ruins of an ancient civilization: *Paradeisos.* Maybe you like the idea of exotic Morocco, with its alluring spices and mysteriously compelling people? *Tagine,* anyone? I could go on and on . . . but perhaps you are starting to see the lay of the land.

Whatever your Mediterranean dream, maybe you, like me, think about this part of the world with longing and wonder because you sense that somehow life is different around that blue-green sun-drenched sea, different than it is here in America. And you would be right . . . in a way. But in another way, you can capture that Mediterranean essence—that lifestyle and that passion—without ever booking passage to Marseille or Valencia or Naples. You can live in the Mediterranean spirit right here, creating the timeless beauty and commonsense joy of living so famously captured in the independent flight of the Venus Winged Victory, the playfulness of Mona Lisa's smile, the classic features of Helen of Troy and Sophia Loren!

What lies ahead for you as you embark on that journey into your own life, attitudes, and kitchen? The journey starts with you, but it will take you to faraway places. No, we won't literally be going anywhere, but in spirit we will be relaxing in the sun and gazing at the sapphire expanse of water to better learn the secrets of that widely varied collection of cultures where women have a rhythm of life, eating, moving, and socializing that isn't quite like anywhere else on the planet. Mediterranean women have a natural vitality, grace, warmth, and earthiness—a style that embodies sensuality, embraces motherhood (*Madonna!*), imparts wisdom, and exudes confidence.

☀ A Trip Around the Sea

The diverse Mediterranean includes Barcelona and Beirut, Algiers and Alexandria, big cities such as Rome and tiny islands such as Crete, Malta, Cyprus, and of course, right at the tip of Italy's boot, Sicily . . . one of my favorite places on Earth.

What can so many cultures have in common, and what can so many different cultures have to teach us? Different as they may be from one another (just as we in America dwell in a nation of cultural diversity), the women living around the Mediterranean Sea do indeed have some secrets that really could change your life for the better. With that in mind, sit back, relax, and get ready to take a brief tour around the Mediterranean. I promise this will be much faster and cheaper than one of those Mediterranean cruises (you know, fourteen days, fourteen countries, just $10,000). Let's look at just how varied the cultures around the Mediterranean really are.

The Mediterranean Sea is much wider than it is long, stretching at its westernmost point from the Strait of Gibraltar, between Spain and Morocco, all the way to Lebanon on the east side. Little pockets here and there have other names. The west coast between Sardinia and Rome is technically the Tyrrhenian Sea. Between the sole and the heel of the boot that is Italy, bordered by Greece on the east side, is the Ionian Sea. And the east coast, between the back of the Italian boot and the land from Croatia to Albania, is the narrow Adriatic Sea. Also, the inlet between Greece and Turkey is the Aegean Sea. But really it's all connected to the Mediterranean, all just divisions of one great sea.

Let's loop around the coastline. We'll start in my favorite spot, the little island of Sicily, smack in the middle of the Mediterranean. Sicily—Palermo is its biggest city—still seems to me to exist in a more ancient time, where people live simply, governed by the weather, the season, and the earth. South of Sicily is another, much smaller island: Malta. Two other little islands, Gozo and Kommuna, nestle up to Malta's main island.

Moving east, you'll find Greece and its myriad tiny islands, including Crete, where the very first study on the Mediterranean diet was based in the 1950s, unveiling to the world that the people of this tiny region were living longer and healthier than anywhere else. Further east you will find the long southern coast of Turkey, with the island of Cyprus just west of Syria's western border. Moving south, you'll find Lebanon, Israel, Jordan, and Egypt, where the Mediterranean Sea feeds the Red Sea (via the Suez Canal) and the Nile River. The northern coasts of Egypt, Libya, and Tunisia (famous for its superspicy cuisine) make up the Mediterranean's southern shore. In the southwest, Algeria cradles Morocco, and with a look north, you'll see Spain. Valencia and Barcelona are the biggest cities on the Mediterranean's far west Spanish coastline, and out into the sea just east of Valencia are the Balearic Islands. Moving north again, France's southern coast, including Marseille, touches the Mediterranean, then we reach gorgeous Monaco. Finally, you'll find northern Italy (just above the islands of Corsica and Sardinia). Almost all of Italy's borders touch the Mediterranean—along the east side, down the west side from Genoa to Rome to Naples, and all the way back south to Sicily again.

✳ The Mediterranean Way of Life

What could all these countries possibly have in common? Just look at where they are located—islands and coastlines all facing one another, all studded with olive trees and grapevines, open-air markets, and relaxed, friendly people with unfurrowed brows and unhurried lifestyles. Life really is different here—

slower, more deliberate, with more presence and attention to the land and each other. You don't see the kind of chronic stress and urban isolation in the Mediterranean that seems to be a common feature of American life. And you don't see the same levels of obesity and overweight, either—at least not among those who still follow the traditional Mediterranean way of life.

That's not to say that every single woman living in the Mediterranean is skinny. Certainly not. People come in all shapes and sizes, with different appetites, activity levels, and genetic predispositions. And in the last decade, rates of obesity all over Europe have risen sharply, especially in children, as eating and lifestyle habits move from traditional Mediterranean ways to American ways that include a sedentary lifestyle and more processed food. The European Union is so concerned about this problem that in March 2005 they launched a new information campaign called Diet, Physical Activity and Health—a European Platform for Action to try to convince people to return to a more traditional Mediterranean lifestyle. In fact, one recent study based in Barcelona showed that the more closely people's diets resembled the traditional Mediterranean diet, the lower their body mass index (a measure of weight and body fat). Conversely, the more they strayed from that traditional diet toward a more "modern" diet, with greater amounts of animal foods and processed foods, fewer fruits and vegetables, and less olive oil, the heavier they were.

What is this traditional Mediterranean diet, lifestyle, and spirit? This book will tell you. It will share the essence of the Mediterranean with you so that you can reap the energizing, slimming, and health-bestowing benefits of this most special way of life. You'll learn how to incorporate fresh, local, seasonal plant food flavored with olive oil and just a little meat into your diet. I eat like this all the time, and you can, too. It's surprisingly easy and mouthwateringly delicious. You'll learn why you need to get up and move more, sit down and eat more, and really wake up and pay attention to your food, your family, and your friends.

You don't need to tour the Mediterranean to learn how to slow down just a little bit and let stress fly out of your life like a helium balloon with a broken string. But you do need to pay attention to your food, breathe deeply, go outside, talk to your friends, be with your family, and (this is important!) learn to *enjoy eating again*.

What better way could there be to lose weight, become slim, feel vibrantly healthy, reclaim your energy, and get back in touch with the earth that produces your food? Eating and living in the spirit of the Mediterranean has nothing to do with deprivation or even willpower. No, this way of life is pure pleasure. You'll learn to take the time to cook for family and friends, to sit down with them for meals and laugh, talk, and eat with relish and passion. Your body will change. Your face will look younger. You'll *feel* younger and maybe even reclaim that waistline you had in your early twenties.

I can practically guarantee that your life will change. Living in contact with the earth, your food, and the people you love will help to coax your best self forward until you feel like your life *is* a Mediterranean vacation. You will find yourself glowing and radiating beauty.

> *In my opinion, there are two things you must recognize about beauty in order to achieve it: first, it is within your reach, and second, it is worth working for.*
>
> **— Sophia Loren, Italian actress**

That's the power of the Mediterranean way of eating, living, and being. Are you with me? Great! Let's begin.

1

Where I Come From

A mild golden sun. An impossibly blue-green sea. A gentle wind like silk with the faint smell of salt. Silver olive trees. Sun-warmed vegetables and fruits ripe to bursting. And people . . . beautiful, friendly, smiling, bright-eyed, contented, healthy, strong, fit people who reach out to help you even if they have no idea who you are. People selling the food they coaxed from the earth. People strolling down the road. People riding their bicycles or sitting in cafes talking and laughing. People in passionate embraces or alone and contemplative, sipping an espresso or choosing a piece of fish at the market or sharing a dessert at an outdoor cafe. Everywhere, people with a sense of place and purpose.

Every time I travel to the Mediterranean, this is the world I experience. In many ways, it seems like a fantasy world to Americans who have never been anywhere near the Mediterranean Sea. Isn't it what we dream of when we imagine an idyllic life without cell phones, laptops, deadlines, meetings, cubicles, recycled office building air, isolation, loneliness, and stress? Don't we fantasize about a world where all those things melt away, where we, too, have calm, smiling faces and strong, slim bodies, and the natural flush of a hard day's physical work . . . and the ability to relax after the work is done?

But this is reality: I can't pick up and move to the Mediterranean. You probably can't, either. At least not anytime soon. But you don't have to, because being *in* the Mediterranean is just one small part of being *of* the Mediterranean. Mediterranean is a lifestyle. An attitude. A spiritual path, if you will. You don't have to live there, and I know because I grew up in that spirit, with that lifestyle and attitude. And I grew up on Long Island.

But even on the east coast of the United States, with the chilly Atlantic as an influence rather than the balmy Mediterranean Sea, the Mediterranean spirit permeated my whole family, which was in many ways governed by my Italian grandfather, Primo Magnani, a butcher by trade and an inveterate gastronome at heart. Primo came to this country from Italy, but instead of taking on America's habits, he clung insistently to his own, passing those along to my mother and right on down to me.

Living in America, *being* an American, but living so fully and wholly in the Mediterranean way, wasn't always easy. But now that I am an adult, living my dream—a Mediterranean dream in which I cook food for others as a profession and actually get paid to do it—*splendido!*—I can see what a difference the Mediterranean lifestyle and attitude has had on my life. At an age when many Americans have been overweight for years, I am not. I feel good, I have energy, and I like the way I look. In typical Mediterranean fashion, however, I don't worry about it too much, either. The Mediterranean lifestyle is about pleasure and passion, feeling good and embracing life. It's about living, right here, right now. The happy side effects, of course, are a slim figure, a strong heart, and a long, healthy life.

That's why I wanted to write this book. You may think that you have to live in the Mediterranean, or at least have Mediterranean ancestry, to really understand and embrace the Mediterranean lifestyle. But nothing could be further from the truth! The Mediterranean lifestyle, at its very essence, is about living wide awake and savoring the pleasures of *region,* of *locality,* of *freshness,* and of the life built around you wherever you live. It doesn't matter if that city is Barcelona or Marseille, San Francisco or St. Louis. No matter where you live, choosing to really live in that place and developing your own connection with your surroundings and the people in them, finding the food that grows there and choosing the very best, learning how to really taste it, getting outside and moving, staying connected with the people who love you . . . now that's living the Mediterranean way.

Every day at my restaurant named after my grandfather Primo, in coastal Maine, I serve food to other people. But I don't get to talk to them as extensively as I would like. I wish I could put ideas on the menu, hints about what it means not just to eat Mediterranean food but to fully embrace the Mediterranean life, where every bite matters, where only the best will do, and where every day is a passionate adventure. In a way, of course, that's what I do by filling the Primo menu with the freshest, best seasonal foods, prepared with love and attention.

In these pages, however, I have more room and more time to share some of my thoughts about what it means to be an American living in the Mediterranean spirit. I want to let you in on some of those secrets that I've discovered from my family, from my travels, and from my grandfather Primo. Let me start by telling you a little bit about my family and how I got to where I am today.

✳ How I Got Here

When I was a kid in school, I felt just a little different, especially in the lunchroom. When other kids took out their bologna sandwiches, potato chips, and Twinkies, I tried to act nonchalant as I opened up my thermos of (how embarrassing) bean and escarole soup. "What's that smell?" my friends would ask, crinkling their noses at the pungent aroma of garlic wafting through the school cafeteria. I clapped the top back on. People just didn't eat like that in America. What was my mother thinking?

I would have done just about anything to bring a lunchbox full of chips and Twinkies to school. No such luck. My mother wasn't about to pack fake food. Once when I was interviewed by the *New York Times*, I mentioned how badly I had wanted to eat Twinkies as a child. That year, my mother sent me a box of Twinkies for Christmas to finally fulfill my decades-long wish. Clever woman that she is, she knew perfectly well that by that point in my life her lessons had stuck, and of course, I wasn't about to eat them.

Now I realize that I was the lucky one. But at the time, although I had plenty of friends and enjoyed school, somehow my Italian family just didn't behave like the other families I knew. It was more than the lunches, but it took me a while to figure out exactly what the differences were. We stood out as we lived and played and worked in our little neighborhood on Long Island. I didn't know then that the way my family was raising me would influence my health, my attitude, my happiness, my ability to love, and even my waistline for the rest of my life.

Our lives were very food centered. My father loved to bake

bread, and my Italian grandmother taught me how to make pasta. We grew up very much in the Italian tradition right across the street from my mom's side of the family. My grandfather Primo taught me a tremendous amount about food. His parents had moved to America from Italy, and food was very important to him. He was this big, robust Italian guy who lived life with gusto. He really knew how to enjoy himself, and his energy infiltrated our entire family as we sat around the dinner table to a traditional meal of soup, a little pasta, fish or meat or sometimes both, and a salad to finish.

We had a garden in the yard, and we went fishing and crabbing all the time. We always had fresh foods and a selection of meats that my grandfather would bring home from the butcher shop where he worked. It was all about the food and gathering the whole family around the table every night to eat, talk, laugh, and eat some more. The funny thing is—and this is only a curiosity if you are entrenched in the American way of eating—that while our table always seemed to overflow with abundance, our bites were little, our portions were small. Meals were about tasting a glorious selection of delicious foods, not about gorging on huge platefuls. An abundant variety tempered with moderation seemed to come naturally to all of us because we didn't know any other way. With tremendous flavors before us, we didn't feel the need to stuff ourselves.

I couldn't help noticing that a lot of my friends sat down to conversationless meals of frozen dinners in front of the television, or ate in shifts, or didn't even know their grandparents, let alone share food, laughter, and time together in the kitchen. In the Mediterranean, mealtime is sacred. Nobody would read a newspaper at the table or eat in shifts or watch television while eating! *Orrible!* And don't even get me started on processed food. It certainly doesn't taste like food to me.

Food fascinates me, and I love it without guilt. I love knowing where it comes from and cooking it in a way that brings out the very best in the ingredients I choose. I eat frequently, and I always enjoy what I eat. I never feel bad about the food on my plate or regret anything I choose to eat. And yet, unlike many Americans, I am slim and healthy. I have never been over-weight. But I don't diet.

What's the secret? Embracing the Mediterranean way of eating, *not* the American way of eating. Embracing a love of food rather than a fear of it. Embracing family, life, and food together in an inseparable and passionate whole. This big picture of eating and living has allowed me to embrace the sensual experience of food and stay at my ideal weight. I eat and live the Mediterranean way.

The best part about eating in the spirit of the Mediterranean is that you don't have to spend six months of every year in Italy, Spain, France, Greece, or Tunisia (nice as that would be) to eat this way. Eating and living in the Mediterranean spirit is equally possible right here in America because it isn't about using a particular kind of fish native only to the Mediterranean Sea or a special spice available only in Greece or a certain type of French cheese. Eating in the Mediterranean style is about the amazing farmers' markets in San Francisco or Manhattan or Madison, Wisconsin. It's about fresh peaches at roadside stands in Georgia or fresh tomatoes and corn on the cob at roadside stands in Iowa. It's about authentic St. Louis barbecue or fish plucked from the waters off the coast of Maine. It's about wild blueberries and you-pick apple orchards and the strawberry patch in your own backyard. It's about where *you* live, and what is fresh right in your own hometown. It's about the people you love and the people who love you, and sharing the full, sensual, aesthetic appreciation of food with community. It's really about living.

The benefits of eating and living this way are not only for

better health, a slimmer figure, and a longer life but for your community as a whole—for your household, your neighborhood, your town or city. If everybody ate only what was produced in their own communities, or at least from their own region of the country, travel would become a special thing indeed rather than the rote exercise of moving from one place to another or the chore of slogging back and forth between here and there. Foreign places would offer special new delights, not the same old stuff shipped to the supermarket from a thousand miles away. And by buying and eating locally, of course, you infuse your own community with energy and resources.

Your community becomes very special when you plumb it for its bounty. You become an expert on seasonality. You know which vegetables are best at what moment, which fruits are ripe, which year has had a good season for apples or grapes, which weather patterns bring out the best in beets or peas. It bothers me that wherever you go in America today, restaurant menus essentially look the same. You can go to San Diego and find fiddlehead ferns and lobster on the menu—specialties of Maine! Likewise, grocery stores on the East Coast often feature produce grown in California. It's all mixed up, and the result is the antithesis of freshness.

✳ My Path to Primo

Before I go on about freshness, as I tend to do, let me tell you a little bit about how I became a chef. I pretty much always worked in the food service industry. In high school, my first job was at a pizzeria. It seemed a natural fit because I was so used to being around food all the time. I continued to work in restaurants during college, then I got a job at a seafood restaurant in Long Island. The chef had graduated from the Culinary Institute of America (CIA) in Hyde Park, New York, and I can't tell you how much I wanted to work in that kitchen. But at that restaurant at that time, there weren't any women in the kitchen. The chef wasn't about to put his reputation on the line by letting untrained me into the inner sanctum of his restaurant, but he told me I should check out the Culinary Institute. If I went to school, he implied, maybe he would hire me. I took this to mean that maybe cooking professionally was something I could do.

So off I went to the Culinary Institute. From that point on, I just fell in love with cooking. I would become a chef, and I knew it. I became very serious and dedicated in school, putting all my energy into learning as much as I could. My favorite part was working in the restaurant at the end of the program, a sort of apprenticeship. Finally, there I was, working in a restaurant kitchen—not the one I'd originally tried to enter but a restaurant kitchen nevertheless. The learning didn't end with school. Every time I travel or even go to a restaurant, I learn something. That's one of the reasons I love food so much. The learning is endless. You never get bored.

I've worked in a lot of restaurants since then, in West Virginia, New York City with Larry Forgione, Miami, and in California at Chez Panisse with Alice Waters, where I really matured as a chef, developing an individual style based on seasonality and freshness, using ingredients from local growers. This is still a big priority for me personally and for Primo, and it really has become a part of my soul. I took this lesson with me when I worked and cooked in Denver, when I traveled to Europe to cook for private families, and even when I went to Japan to help open a restaurant. By the time I was hired at Old Chatham Sheepherding Company Inn in the beautiful Hudson Valley (New York), I felt I had truly come full circle back to my roots, embracing a true calling.

Old Chatham Sheepherding Company is the largest sheep dairy farm in America, with more than a thousand sheep. They milk the sheep and make wonderful cheese. When I was hired, the farm had an old house on the property, and they wanted to open a bed-and-breakfast. They said they were looking for a chef, but I didn't want to be limited to cooking breakfast, so I talked them into having a restaurant along with the inn. My partner, Price, and I ran it for four and a half years. I was the chef and Price was the pastry chef. We had an innkeeper, we put in a garden, and we cooked from the garden and had lambs and pigs on the premises for use in the kitchen. We had a big budget and it was a great experience, but we knew all along that what we really wanted was to open our own restaurant. We got all kinds of accolades for the work we did and the food we cooked. But Price and I had our eyes on Maine.

The beauty of the Maine coast really drew us there. Price's parents owned property in Rockland. Finding a 125-year-old Victorian house just outside of town on four lovely acres seemed to be a good sign. That was in 1999. The house was stuffy, with layers of wall coverings and heavy carpet. We didn't have a lot of money, so we decided to do all the renovation ourselves. We stripped the house to its bare bones, then let it breathe—a metaphor for the way I like to prepare food. It took eight months, but the house became fresh. It was open and alive again.

And we've been here ever since. Freshness is our mantra at Primo and the guiding principle behind everything we do. I change Primo's menu every single day to feature what I can get right here, right now. Only our field green salad, which we call Lucy's Salad after our head grower, Lucy Yanz, and our seasonal pizza, remain on the menu, although they change in composition according to the season. Primo's menu is ultimately seasonal with a Mediterranean flavor. I grow most of the ingredients we use right here on Primo's grounds. During parts of the year, the restaurant is almost totally self-sustaining.

We make our own vinegar, we grow our own organic herbs, we have a tea garden, and we have huge vegetable and flower gardens on the grounds. Lucy nurtures them all. We also have two greenhouses where we grow winter greens all year, and one greenhouse stays warm in the dead of winter even though it is unheated. Price makes his own sourdough starter, which he feeds three times a day to keep it alive for the most wonderful bread filled with energy and life. We even raise pigs and buy local chickens for use in the restaurant. We butcher on the premises, make our own stock, and use only the seafood we can get right here from the waters off the coast.

✳ A New Way to Eat

Sometimes, the food I serve at Primo is a hard sell for Americans. It's really a whole new way for many people to eat. People love chicken, but they aren't sure they want to try rabbit. They love halibut but are hesitant about wolffish, even though this local delicacy is delicious. The wolffish in Maine eat the lobster and crab in the local water, so their meat is white and sweet, yet much less expensive than lobster or halibut. Wolffish live 5,000 feet deep in the water, where it is supercold, so they have an incredibly clean taste. Also, wolffish is not overcooked like halibut and cod. Everyone who tries this fish loves it. But many people don't like to try anything new. That's one habit that everyone should break! Healthy eating must include variety.

People often ask me about how I stay so thin as a chef. I taste food all day long, but that is part of the key to my way of eating. I'm very conscious of everything I eat. I pay attention to my food because food is so important to me—because I love food so much. I don't mindlessly shove food into my mouth, because that would be such a terrible waste not only of food but of my own essential vitality. I would miss out on the goodness.

In the morning, I usually eat a little yogurt or granola. I drink tea all day long, and I eat a lot of vegetables, nuts, and fruits, the bulk of my diet. I have balance in my diet. I really work for that because of the way it makes me feel and because that is how I have learned to eat. When I eat protein such as fish or meat, I have a small portion, maybe 4 ounces, not a 12-ounce steak. Because I am always tasting, tasting, tasting, I have a lot of little meals throughout the day.

Research backs up this approach to eating. A recent study compared two groups of people eating the same number of calories every day. One group ate all the calories in two meals. The other ate the same number of calories but in five little meals. After twelve weeks, the group eating twice per day lost weight, but evaluations revealed it was primarily muscle weight. The group eating more meals also lost weight, and it was almost entirely weight from fat! When you are trying to keep your metabolism up and your body burning fat throughout the day, little tastes are definitely the way to go. It's the body's natural way to snack rather than stuff.

Sure, sometimes I get really hungry. But when I do, I don't grab chips or those Twinkies I used to think I wanted so badly. I make a beautiful salad or crunch some fresh vegetables from the garden outside the door, or I snack on a handful of nuts. Let me give you an example of some of the things I might snack on—Mediterranean classic tastes that are most assuredly *not* junk food but are perfectly wonderful as snack food. These are simple to make, easy to eat, and convenient to have with you when you get hungry.

Spicy Walnuts

These spicy walnuts really wake up the palate. You don't need too many, but a handful of nuts each day has been linked to good heart health. Exercising Mediterranean restraint, enjoy a few of these meaty, spicy nuts as a prelude to your family dinner or when you have hunger pangs between meals.

4 tablespoons unsalted butter

1/2 teaspoon cayenne pepper

2 teaspoons prepared Cajun seasoning
(or combine 1/2 teaspoon each
minced garlic, coriander, hot
paprika, and onion powder)

2 teaspoons ground cumin

3 tablespoons sugar

1 pound raw walnuts, large pieces

Salt to taste

1. In a medium saucepan over medium heat, melt the butter until it foams. Add the cayenne pepper, Cajun seasoning, cumin, and sugar, and mix well.

2. Add the walnuts and toss until toasted and just starting to darken in color, about 5 minutes. Spread the walnuts on a cooling rack over a tray or baking sheet to cool. Dust with salt and serve. Store remaining nuts in an airtight container up to 3 weeks.

Olive Sampler

If you don't like olives, you may have never tried the really good kind from the Mediterranean. I don't mean those green, pimiento-stuffed "Spanish" olives (really from California) that are better off in somebody's martini. I mean small French picholines or niçoise olives, plump kalamata olives from Greece, Spanish Arbequina olives, salt-cured olives from North Africa . . . and that's just the beginning. Olives have such an intense flavor that you only need a few to feel like you've really tasted something. Fortunately, most grocery store delis offer a variety of good Mediterranean olives.

The best way to get to know olives is to try them. Pick up a jar of assorted olives the next time you are at the market, or get several small containers of different kinds. Be careful of the pits! Most Mediterranean olives still have them, but they are easy to remove. Just whack the olive with the flat side of a chef's knife, then pop out the pit with your fingers. Each type of olive has its unique taste, texture, and color. Learn to appreciate olives, and you'll have a new ingredient to incorporate into your cooking. You'll also have a quick snack to wake up your palate.

Some people may worry about the high fat content of olives, but this is no more of a concern than the fat content of olive oil. Olives are part of the Mediterranean diet that results in better health and lower weight: Mediterranean olives have such intense flavor that just a few are satisfying. Plus, they contain the same heart-healthy oil as olive oil (you'll learn all about this in chapter 4), so eating olives is just one more way to make olive oil the primary source of fat in your diet. Snacking on a few olives is like snacking on a handful of nuts: they are filling and satisfying. So enjoy those savory olives!

Another way to enjoy olives is to add them to a salad. Combine fresh greens, a handful of olives, a handful of fresh almonds, some chopped fresh tomatoes, a drizzle of extra-virgin olive oil, and freshly squeezed lemon juice. That should take care of your hunger pangs.

Cheese Sampler

Cheese is another great snack for satisfying your hunger, but you don't need a lot of it. Forget bland American cheese (or worse yet, "cheese food"!). Mediterranean cheese is often made from sheep's milk or goat's milk, and any store with a respectable gourmet cheese section will offer at least a few good-quality cheeses from the Mediterranean. Some are for cooking, such as creamy ricotta; others are for grating, such as Parmesan, pecorino, and Romano. Today there are great American cheese makers producing Mediterranean-quality cheeses. Buy locally!

You can also enjoy cheese out of hand or on a salad, a toasted pita wedge, or a thin slice of baguette. Try Greek feta, French Roquefort or Camembert, Italian Gorgonzola, Spanish Manchego—these are just a few of the hundreds of Mediter-ranean cheeses available. Many American dairies and artisanal cheese makers produce beautiful, delicious fresh cheese from sheep's milk and goat's milk, including my favorite (and former employer), Old Chatham Sheepherding Company. Look for American-made artisinal versions of your favorite cheese styles. Ask the person at the cheese or deli counter what's new, what's good, what to try. If you always have at least two different wedges of high-quality cheese in your house, you'll never go hungry.

Fruit Mélange

What could be sweeter than a perfectly ripe piece of fruit? In the Mediterranean, fruit is dessert, but it is also something to eat when you need a snack between meals. Eating a ripe piece of fruit is an event in itself in the sensual Mediterranean, where the firm, ripe flesh, the flowing juice, and the round curve of a perfect fruit suggest pure pleasure. We often refrigerate our fruits, which hinders the juiciness somewhat and impedes flavor, all to be able to keep the fruit around longer. Fruit should be kept on the counter and eaten when it can barely hold its juices any longer. What luxury. Certainly you are perfectly fulfilled after eating a snack like that! Don't you feel just a little more Mediterranean already?

✳ Stepping into the Mediterranean Spirit

Whenever I visit Sicily, I am struck by how similar it is to Maine. Both look out over the sea. Both are a little old-fashioned yet in so being, they become almost progressive. In big cities, everybody is striving to imitate the old ways. Sicily is still steeped in the old ways that Americans want to reclaim so desperately.

In Sicily, people really do go to the market every day. You can wander through the stands and stalls and meet a little, old Sicilian lady standing on the side of the street filleting anchovies. You can ask to take her picture, and she is so happy to pose for you and smile. In Sicily, people love what they do. They are proud and they love their lives. Life is very food centered, so it seems that almost everything people do is somehow linked to nourishment. For instance, they really appreciate the antipasto part of the meal. I grew up with this tradition in my own family. Meals began with these great platters of delicious bits of cooked grains, marinated vegetables, salads, and dips for vegetables. It was really more about the social coming together of the family than anything. It was about sitting around the table with your friends and family and eating things that please you. In Sicily, they still participate in that savory tradition.

One of the reasons I love to visit Spain so much is because of the huge variety. They serve lots of different plates, each full of flavor, and they are so much more adventurous about what they will try, from unusual vegetables to seafood many Americans have never heard of before. All over the Mediterranean, women eat so many more different kinds of vegetables and fruits and meats and especially seafood, things we either can't get or, more often, would never dare to try. But can't we all use a little bit more daring in our diets? A little more excitement? More flavor and sensuality?

Lots of little dishes are great because you can turn the leftovers into something else. Chickpeas in your salad one day become a dip the next day. Leftover vegetables become part of an antipasto or a meze platter. This transformation of leftovers is fun and convenient—cooking enough on one day to make three days of delicious meals.

In the Mediterranean, particularly in the smallest towns and villages, life is still very basic. The women and their families with whom I talked are perfectly happy to live apart from the rush and stress of the city. They have enough to do. Their lives are enough, and that's how I feel about my life here in Maine. That's how I feel about my life as a whole, the way I have built it and the way I live it. This is how I stay slim, healthy, and happily satisfied with my busy—but not too busy—life.

Anyone can find this same pace and learn deep in her own soul how to eat and live the Mediterranean way. Imagine what your world would be like if you slowed down, paid attention, and embraced every moment of sensual pleasure. Imagine knowing exactly where every bite of food you put in your mouth came from. Imagine feeling with ultimate clarity how the food you eat affects your body and letting your body's wisdom guide your choices. Imagine your body glowing with vibrant health and energy. Imagine feeling happy, slim, content, loved.

In this book, I lay out all the components of living and eating in the style of the Mediterranean, including the most luscious and wonderful recipes that will help you take full advantage of your local resources, live wide awake, and really taste and enjoy every bite of food. These are the keys to energy and health. If you need to lose weight, you will. You will feel better. You will lessen your risk of disease. You may even live longer. And I can practically guarantee you will look more beautiful.

One of my favorite Italian sayings is *A tavola non si invecchia*—"At the table, one never grows old." At a table with good food, good friends, a loving family, and an abundant variety of fresh, locally grown food, I would also add that while a woman might easily fill up on passion, she need never grow fat.

> *There is no end. There is no beginning. There is only the infinite passion of life.*
> **—Federico Fellini, Italian film director**

It's all part of *la dolce vita*, the sweet life, the Mediterranean life, and a whole new yet magnificently ancient key to life, health, and the body you've always wanted.

2

Good Taste

THE SLIMMING POWER OF HIGH FLAVOR

Food and life are inextricably linked. Aristotle, the most famous Mediterranean philosopher, wrote, "To nurture the soul is to feed it." I couldn't agree more. Right at the crossroads where food and the soul meet is vitality, meaning energy, good health, good feeling, a spiritual connection to your life, and a body you feel good to be inside.

What are you feeding your soul? Aristotle wrote these words in 350 B.C., proving how essential the food–life link has been for thousands of years in the Mediterranean. To nurture the soul is to feed it, and to feed the body well is to nurture the soul. In the Mediterranean, the symbiosis of eating and being has evolved through the centuries to produce the most healthful and diverse diet on the planet. But knowing about it isn't enough. Eating a salad now and then isn't enough. You have to embrace vitality in all its facets. This chapter asks you to consider how well you feed your soul, how much you understand about your relationship with food, and how you can go about improving that relationship so that you can stay or get slim.

> **The beginning is the half of every action.**
> **— Greek proverb**

✳ Your One-Day, Three-Step Pleasure-Eating Meditation

What do you eat? Do you even know? Mindless eating is a common habit, and most Americans do it to some extent. I see entire families mindlessly eating all the time. Women eat on the go just like they put their makeup on while driving. They eat while watching television, or walking to work. Women eat while sitting in front of their computers, surfing the Internet for entertainment, or they snack while working at the computers in their offices. A lot of women spend their lunch hour working and eating at the same time.

I admit to having an advantage here. I eat all day long because I am forced to taste food and really pay attention as part of my job. If I'm sampling dishes we are going to serve at Primo that night, I'd better be paying attention! I don't want to serve food that is bland, boring, or bad. I want what I serve to be fresh, bright, and deliciously alive in the mouth. If that's not what I get, I start over again.

But for most American women, noticing what they eat isn't nearly so easy. My three-step process will let taste work for you. Contrary to what you may think, really wonderful tastes help you eat less, not more. When we eat, we seek energy, of course, but we also seek pleasure. When our pleasure is fulfilled, we are fulfilled and can stop eating. But if we aren't getting pleasure from our food, we keep on eating (searching) to find that pleasure. And we eat too much.

The other thing that happens is that we eat while getting "pleasure" (or at least a distraction) from something else. The problem is that we miss the opportunity to get pleasure from our food, which is such a life-sustaining source of pleasure, and we tend to eat too much. You know what I mean. Surely you've been sitting in front of the television eating a bag of potato chips and suddenly you realize the whole thing is gone. Where did all the chips go? Didn't you just have about four servings there in front of you? You consumed calories and fat you didn't need and you didn't even get to enjoy it because you were too busy paying attention to something else. Is this feeding your soul?

Back to the three-step process. I want you to try something for one day. Just one day. Just to see how it sits with you. This one-day plan isn't hard, but you may struggle with it because it isn't the way you are used to doing things. Consider it your One-Day, Three-Step Pleasure-Eating Meditation. That doesn't sound so bad, does it? Every time you eat, I want you to:

1. Stop doing everything else.
2. Focus totally on the taste of every single bite.
3. Chew every bite thirty times.

Let's look at what these steps really mean for you.

Step 1: Stop Doing Everything Else

If you stop doing everything else, the only thing you are doing is eating. No eating while reading the newspaper or a magazine or even a really great novel. (One pleasure at a time, please!) No eating at your desk at work if you are even looking at any of your work. No talking on the phone while you eat or listening to music. Turn everything off. Take the phone off the hook. If you are at work, leave your desk and go outside or perhaps to the lobby. Or get in the car and drive somewhere. (But no eating while driving!) Or just turn your chair away from that pile of work.

To make this step easier when you are at home, you can designate a spot for eating. Did you ever consider the dining room table? Clear it off and reserve it for your one day. Whenever you eat anything—even a bite, even a taste of something—go to that spot, sit down, breathe, relax, and focus.

What about your partner, your children, your coworkers? Sure, you can eat with them. They are eating, too. You can talk to your family, but when you take a bite of your food, taste it. Talk about it! See what the other people in your life think about the taste. Don't talk about anything else while you are actually eating—just talk about the food.

Step 2: Focus Totally on the Taste of Every Single Bite

Now for the pleasure part. Since you've eliminated all distractions, I want you to pay attention. Look at your plate. Look at the food. Notice the color, the texture, the aroma. Take a big whiff. It's okay to go, "Ahhhhh!" This is your pleasure day, remember?

Now take a bite. Take a long, slow, languorous bite. Really taste what you are eating. Feel the texture in your mouth, the flavor, the way the aroma mingles with the taste . . . revel in the whole experience.

Just imagine eating like this all the time! Guess who does that? Yes, Mediterranean women.

Step 3: Chew Every Bite Thirty Times

Chewing is an important part of good digestion. Gulping down your food sends it into your body before it is ready. Not only do you stress your digestion, but you miss out on a lot of the pleasure. Once the food is out of contact with your taste buds, the experience of that one beautiful bite begins to fade. So make it last. Chew slowly, savor the food, and only swallow when you've chewed at least thirty times.

I understand that some food doesn't require much chewing, and you may not be able to chew it thirty times. Just consider it a goal to see how long you can keep each pleasurable bite in your mouth.

Follow these three steps for every single bite of food you take for one full day. Believe me, you'll be more satisfied by your meals and you'll eat less food. Who can argue with those results?

If you followed these steps for one day, couldn't you possibly do it for two days? Or three? How about for most of the meals you enjoy for the rest of your life? Now you're eating in the Mediterranean spirit!

What if the taste experience is unpleasant? What if you eat something you thought you liked and suddenly it doesn't taste very good? Maybe it isn't very fresh or crisp or juicy, or maybe you detect a chemical taste (common in processed food to those paying attention to taste). Maybe you just think the food is boring. Then don't eat it! Push it aside. If someone else is serving the food, just say that you are full. *J'ai mangé à ma faim, merci.* When it comes to taste, I give you full permission to be a food snob. Your body deserves only the very best.

✳ Little Tastes of Big Flavor

In the Mediterranean, food is both seasonal and unprocessed, not only because that is what is available but because seasonal, fresh food tastes so much better. You wouldn't eat asparagus in the winter, peaches in late fall, apples in the spring. And canned peaches? Only if you canned them yourself using peaches from your local market! While processed food has become more popular in some parts of the Mediterranean (that trend toward "Americanization"), in small villages along the sea and in places such as Sicily, the notion of canned food and tasteless frozen dinners would seem absurd.

Taste is the essential focus of the Mediterranean diet. But the palate is a funny thing. You would think that foods taste a certain way to everyone; however, taste doesn't seem to work that way at all. Instead, the palate is ever-changing, ever-evolving, and every palate is a little different. What your mouth appreciates may be directly related to your past experiences, so what you like may be completely different than what I like. What I taste, even in a simple dish such as minted yogurt or tomatoes with fresh tarragon, may be different than what you taste.

For people who aren't used to strong, bright, clear flavors, Mediterranean cuisine may feel like an adjustment. Is food really supposed to have that much taste? Is it supposed to be so passionately intense in its color, texture, and flavor? *Sí, señora!* If you are used to bland, overly salted, processed food, canned vegetables and fruit, or only a few basic tastes in your everyday eating, then you are in for a treat! You won't believe healthy eating can be this seductive.

The more you sample and savor flavors you've never tried before and taste combinations that are new to you, the more your palate will learn to get excited by new sensations. If your palate is used to potato chips or processed "diet" foods, well . . . maybe it's time to broaden your palate's experience.

I was lucky enough to start eating high-flavor food as a child, but some of you may not be used to this kind of eating. You might wrinkle your nose at the strong smell of garlic or the concentrated tang of sun-dried tomatoes. Or maybe you think these tastes are thrilling, or hope they will be. Now is the time to start discovering, testing, and challenging your own palate.

In this chapter, we will look at and taste some of the most basic flavors of Mediterranean cuisine. This is way beyond salt and pepper, mayonnaise and ketchup, my friends. This is garlic and lemon, parsley and mint, tart yogurt and sweet balsamic vinegar, toasted coriander and cumin. This is flavor.

The cooking part won't be difficult at all. If you aren't used to cooking much beyond your microwave, don't worry. I may be a chef, but I know how it is to be crunched for time, hungry, and standing in the middle of your kitchen without fancy equipment and gourmet ingredients. We'll start with some very simple recipes to introduce your palate to new flavors. And we'll talk about the best ways to get the most out of your meal so that you learn not only what to taste but how to taste.

As we venture forth into a world of new, powerful, vibrant, exciting tastes, we will first experiment with a few very basic tastes characteristic of Mediterranean cuisine, highlighted in a few simple recipes. These aren't meals. These little dishes make excellent bites to experiment with on your One-Day, Three-Step Pleasure-Eating Meditation because you can be assured of high flavor with a Mediterranean character.

I will suggest some simple ways you can use these tastes to add excitement to the foods you probably eat every day: chicken, pasta, tuna, salad, bread. Chicken soup sprinkled with gremolata is fresher, brighter, and more intense than plain chicken soup. A bowl of pasta tossed with red pesto is much more interesting than pasta with canned tomato sauce, and a thin slice of toasted baguette tastes a lot better with buttery roasted garlic spread across it than plain butter. Are you ready to taste with me? Let's get into the kitchen.

Garlic

Remember my thermos of bean and escarole soup? That soup was redolent with rich, aromatic garlic. Garlic is one of the most ancient vegetables on the planet, and many cuisines all over the globe use it as an integral flavoring component. Garlic can taste pungent and eye-wateringly strong or mellow, rich, and heady with flavor—it all depends on what you do with it. Raw garlic can be spicy. It has a little zing with a light sauté. Cooked golden brown, it has a toasted, earthy flavor, slow-roasted, it becomes sweet and mellow with a velvety texture. Rub a clove on a toasted crostini and the crumb of the bread will grate the garlic into the crevices.

When your palate gets used to the taste of garlic, you can begin to recognize its presence in many different dishes. Garlic is one of the key tastes in Mediterranean cuisine. Even in ancient Rome, people thought garlic had healing powers and used it therapeutically for everything from treating topical infections as an antiseptic to curing asthma. They were right. Raw garlic can kill bacteria, fungus, yeast, and when it is cooked, it has a blood-thinning effect that can help lower blood pressure and cholesterol levels and even open up clogged arteries. It also contains a host of phytochemicals that may have a potent anti-cancer effect.

But garlic's stellar qualities aside, it has a most wonderful taste and aroma, which is probably why it is a common ingredient in many classic Mediterranean dishes, from soups and stews to braises, sauces, marinades, and salad dressings. When you cook garlic the right way, it tastes buttery and flavorful but mellow—you might not believe it's garlic. I'm going to show you how to enjoy garlic in this wonderful way, and it could hardly be simpler.

Tasting roasted garlic on bread will help your palate memorize garlic's flavor so that you can recognize it and feel more confident using it in your own cooking. You may never want to put butter on your bread again. Spread it on slices of baguette with a little cheese, then broil for a few minutes to make luscious garlic-cheese bread. Try it on crackers, cucumber slices, or thin slices of Roma tomatoes. Or use it on a sandwich for a quick and flavorful lunch. Try this simple recipe: Spread roasted garlic on a slice of bread, then top with a freshly sliced tomato. Sprinkle on freshly chopped basil, a teaspoon of freshly grated Parmesan cheese, and freshly ground black pepper.

> *Tomatoes and oregano make it Italian; wine and tarragon make it French. Sour cream makes it Russian; lemon and cinnamon make it Greek. Soy sauce makes it Chinese; garlic makes it good.*
>
> —Alice May Brock, writer

Roasted Garlic

Choose a bulb of garlic that looks plump and large, with firm cloves. If it feels soft or has green sprouts, the garlic is old and no good. A mild Spanish olive oil is good for this recipe, but any quality extra-virgin olive oil will work.

1 garlic bulb (not just a clove)
1–2 teaspoons extra-virgin olive oil

8 thin baguette slices, or 4 Italian bread slices

1. Preheat the oven to 400°F. Slice off just the top quarter inch of the garlic bulb, exposing the tops of all the cloves.

2. Set the garlic cut side up in a pie plate and drizzle with olive oil, making sure you get some oil on all the garlic cloves. Bake for about 30 minutes. Let the garlic cool just enough that you can handle it.

3. Toast the slices of bread. Squeeze the garlic paste from the cloves (the soft garlic paste should slip easily from the skins), or scoop it out with a small spoon, and spread it on the toast. Slowly savor the taste of garlic the way it is meant to be eaten.

Agrodolce

Agrodolce means "sour-sweet," and this is a classic taste combination in Mediterranean food. Many vegetables can be prepared agrodulce. Fish also tastes good this way. The sour usually comes from vinegar or lemon juice, while the sweet may be from balsamic vinegar, currants, raisins, honey, or sugar. This taste combination may be foreign to you, but try this classic Mediterranean preparation to introduce your palate to this essential taste experience. Cooking vegetables this way might just help you eat more of them. You can snack on them at room temperature or even straight out of the refrigerator if you don't have time to warm them up.

Cipollini Agrodolce

Serves 2

Cipollini onions are Italian baby onions, but you can substitute any small onion in this dish, such as pearl onions; or use sweet Vidalia onions if they are freshly available, and slice them thinly. You want mild, sweet onions for this dish rather than big pungent onions. If you don't have access to onions, you can try this dish with another mild vegetable such as eggplant, peeled and cut into small cubes, or even zucchini. Use whatever is freshest.

1 tablespoon extra-virgin olive oil
1 cup peeled and sliced Cipolline or
    other small, sweet onions
1/2 teaspoon salt
Freshly ground black pepper
    to taste
1 tablespoon honey

1 tablespoon chopped fresh thyme
    or 1 teaspoon dried thyme
1 bay leaf
2 cinnamon sticks, or 1/4 teaspoon
    ground cinnamon
1/2 teaspoon sherry vinegar or other
    good-quality wine vinegar

1. Preheat the oven to 400°F. Heat the olive oil in a medium ovenproof sauté pan over medium-high heat. When you can smell the oil (after about 2 minutes), add the onions. Sear the onions, stirring constantly.

2. When the onions turn soft and brown and start to caramelize, add the salt, pepper, and honey. Toss to coat. Continue to cook and stir for about 3 more minutes, then remove the pan from the heat.

3. Stir in the thyme, bay leaf, and cinnamon. Place the pan in the oven. Bake the onion mixture for 10 minutes.

4. Stir in the vinegar. Remove the bay leaf and cinnamon sticks, and serve warm or at room temperature.

Olives

Olive trees decorate the Mediterranean. Their fruit is absolutely essential to Mediterranean cuisine. Since ancient times, people have kept great vats of olive oil. It's a key component in Mediterranean cuisine and the source of most of the fat in the Mediterranean diet. This kind of fat is good for your heart. I've devoted a whole chapter to olive oil (chapter 4). But for now, let's consider the humble olive itself and its distinctive taste.

One recipe I really enjoy is tapenade. This is a spreadable black olive paste uniquely flavored with tangy capers and salty anchovies. Don't be afraid to use anchovies—they are a key taste component of tapenade and are a frequent flavoring in many Mediterranean dishes. Most grocery stores carry them. Anchovies aren't obvious in many recipes, and if you didn't know the recipe included anchovies, you probably wouldn't be able to guess by the taste. But they do add that *je ne sais quoi.* Tapenade tastes good on toasted or grilled slices of bread, crackers, or even as a sandwich spread. Try it as an interesting alternative the next time you feel like enjoying a tuna salad sandwich. Tapenade is so rich and flavorful that you only need a little to feel satisfied.

Tapenade

Makes about 2½ cups

Tapenade should be slightly chunky, not a completely smooth paste. You should be able to see grain-sized bits of olives, but the mixture should be easily spreadable. Pitting the olives isn't hard—you can almost consider it a meditative act. Whack each olive with the side of a chef's knife, then just pop out the pit with your fingers by squeezing the olive. For a nuttier flavor, try this with Sicilian green olives or fleshy Greek olives.

2 cups pitted kalamata olives

1½ tablespoons chopped garlic, or a little more if needed

3 tablespoons capers

4 fresh or canned anchovy fillets, rinsed and patted dry

¼ cup fresh basil leaves, or more if needed

1 tablespoon extra-virgin olive oil, or a little more if needed

1 teaspoon freshly squeezed lemon juice, or more if needed

1. Puree all the ingredients together in a food processor until combined but still textured. If the tapenade is too stiff or not spreadable, stir in a little more olive oil.

2. Taste and adjust the seasonings, adding more garlic, basil, or lemon juice if necessary, or even a pinch of sea salt. Store in a glass jar in the refrigerator for up to 1 week.

Parsley-Garlic-Citrus and Other Herb-Spice Combos

In Mediterranean cooking, certain herb and spice combinations give foods a classic taste profile. Italy, France, Spain, Greece, North Africa—each has its distinctive taste combinations, and learning what these are will help you make basic food more interesting and any food more exotic and Mediterranean in taste. Mediterranean herb-spice combinations are typically so vibrant and forward in their tastes that they are a great way to help you eat less and enjoy your food more. They make every bite more delightful.

• •

To capture the flavor of different Mediterranean countries, just add the right herb-spice-condiment combo. Here's what to add to your favorite dish of pasta or bland piece of chicken or fish to give it Mediterranean flair:

- For Moroccan flavor, try cinnamon, walnuts, raisins, cloves
- For French flavor, try the herb blend called herbes de Provence, which includes marjoram, thyme, savory, basil, rosemary, sage, lavender, and a little fennel seed
- For Spanish flavor, try saffron, white onion, sage, rosemary, smoked or hot paprika
- For Italian flavor, try oregano, basil, thyme, olives, capers, sweet peppers, garlic, tomatoes, dried pepperoncini
- For Greek flavor, add lemon, feta cheese, olives, capers, or mint, honey, yogurt, oregano
- For Tunisian flavor, try harissa (a spicy condiment made with hot chile peppers) and curry
- For North African flavor, add paprika, garlic, ginger, chiles, raisins, sweet potatoes, cumin, coriander, dried ground rose petals

• •

Many combinations contain fresh parsley—the flat-leaf kind marked "Italian parsley" at the market. Often combined with citrus rind and garlic, parsley can be cooked into dishes or chopped and sprinkled raw over the top of meat, fish, or vegetables. One of the classic ways to use parsley in Mediterranean cooking is in gremolata, an Italian flavoring mixture that is usually sprinkled over cooked food right before serving, adding a bright, fresh taste and making bland food more exciting. Typically a mixture of chopped parsley, garlic, and lemon rind, gremolata is the traditional garnish for osso buco, the delicious veal shank stew that is itself an Italian classic.

Try using parsley in your cooking more often. Use my gremolata recipe for garnishing, or try it over soup or stew to add a Mediterranean flair. Spread it on a chicken breast before grilling. Sprinkle it over halibut for an elegant dinner, or mix it with canned tuna and stuff into half a whole-wheat pita for an elegant but quick lunch.

Gremolata

This version of gremolata uses orange rind instead of lemon, but you can use either one. The delicious flavor of toasted coriander seeds—the seeds that grow the cilantro plant—add depth. Use Italian parsley in this dish rather than curly parsley. You can also add mint or anise hyssop.

3 tablespoons coriander seeds
Zest of 3 oranges (reserve fruit for another use)
2 cups chopped fresh Italian parsley

2 tablespoons extra-virgin olive oil
½ teaspoon salt
2 garlic cloves, peeled and finely minced

1. Heat a small skillet over medium-high heat and toast the coriander seeds, stirring constantly, until they turn just a shade darker brown and you start to smell them. This should take just 2–3 minutes. Remove from the heat. Be careful not to burn them. If you burn any, just throw those away.

2. Thoroughly combine the toasted coriander seeds with the other ingredients in a medium bowl. Store in a glass jar in the refrigerator for up to 4 days.

Yogurt and Mint

Classic Mediterranean food doesn't include a lot of dairy, but certain cheeses are used, and in some countries, a lot of yogurt. If you aren't used to yogurt or you are only used to the kind of yogurt that you buy in the grocery store premixed with a bunch of sugary fruit, then you haven't really tried yogurt Mediterranean style—yogurt that is creamy, rich, and tangy. The natural probiotics in yogurt help keep your digestion in good working order, which can be a great help if you are eating more vegetables and grains.

In the Mediterranean, yogurt is usually used in savory dishes rather than sweet dishes. I love the taste of plain yogurt, but you might not be used to it yet. Experiment with it. Use the whole-milk variety, and relish that rich, creamy texture and mouth-filling taste. Use yogurt in recipes that call for sour cream or crème fraîche. Eat one spoonful every day. Add a teaspoon of maple syrup—it's delicious! Pretty soon you'll be hooked.

Another way people use yogurt in the Mediterranean is to drain it in a colander lined with cheesecloth so that it becomes thick, like the consistency of whipped cream cheese. This yogurt spread or yogurt cheese is great as a sandwich spread with fresh vegetables on good bread, and you can even make cheesecake with it. Mix it with fresh fruit and spread it on toast, or slather it on pita bread and top it with white beans, chopped tomatoes, and slivers of fresh basil.

You can buy some really good yogurt in the store these days. Goat's milk and sheep's milk yogurt are very authentic for the Mediterranean. If you're interested, yogurt is simple to make with a basic yogurt maker that keeps the milk at just the right temperature to become yogurt. These machines make about 1 quart at a time, keeping you supplied with fresh yogurt all week. I like the inexpensive Salton machine, which makes yogurt in a single quart container. It is easy to use and clean.

Mint is another popular herb in Mediterranean cooking, particularly in Greece. Mint sauce is a classic accompaniment to lamb. People like to flavor peas and potatoes with mint, but I like to put it in yogurt. Mint grows like a weed in most climates, so it is easy to have fresh mint on hand. Freeze or dry extra mint for year-round use. Try this recipe to see if it doesn't help win you over to yogurt's savory side.

Mint Yogurt

This recipe combines plain yogurt with herbs and spices. Mint yogurt is delicious as a garnish on a simple bowl of chickpea or white bean soup, or as a condiment on a sandwich of chicken or lamb wrapped in warm pita bread. Or just eat it with a spoon.

1 cup plain yogurt
2 tablespoons chopped fresh mint
2 tablespoons chopped fresh cilantro
1 teaspoon minced garlic
1/4 teaspoon ground cumin

Freshly ground black pepper to taste
1/2 teaspoon salt
1 tablespoon freshly squeezed lime
*   juice*

1. Combine all the ingredients in a small bowl.

2. Cover and chill for at least 1 hour so that the flavors can blend. Serve chilled. Store in the refrigerator for up to 1 week.

Salsa

Salsa is the Spanish word for sauce. Although we usually associate salsa with Mexican cuisine, it is an important part of Spanish cuisine, too. Salsa usually refers to an uncooked sauce or relish that is often spicy. A variety of salsas make great accompaniments to fresh vegetables. Salsas are so much better tasting and better for you than fatty, bland dressings and dips. They are also quick and easy to make. Just put two cloves of peeled garlic, one teaspoon sea salt, and two to four cored and seeded hot chile peppers (like jalapeños) in a food processor. Pulse a few times to chop. Add four cored fresh tomatoes and a cored and seeded green or red bell pepper. Puree. Stir in one-quarter cup chopped fresh cilantro and the juice from one lime and voilà! Fresh salsa.

Salsa verde simply means "green sauce," and it is the Italian version of salsa, using Italian herbs: parsley, capers, anchovies, lemon, and olive oil. It's nothing at all like the tomato salsa you are used to, but try it for a change and relish the bright, bold flavor.

Salsa Verde

Try this recipe with toasted pita bread, grilled baguette slices, as a garnish for cooked foods, or even stirred into freshly cooked hot pasta. Or split open a baguette, sprinkle the inside with a good sherry vinegar, spread this salsa on both sides, and share with a friend. If you include the hard-boiled eggs, you've got lunch. Use whatever herbs are freshly available in addition to the parsley.

¾ cup chopped fresh Italian parsley

¼ cup chopped fresh basil, oregano, chives, and/or rosemary

¼ cup capers

2 fresh or canned anchovy fillets, rinsed, patted dry, and chopped

1 tablespoon Dijon mustard

1 teaspoon freshly squeezed lemon juice

1 tablespoon extra-virgin olive oil

½ teaspoon salt

Freshly ground black pepper to taste

2 hard-boiled eggs, chopped (optional)

1. Combine all the ingredients in a medium bowl.

2. Let the salsa sit for at least 1 hour so that the flavors can blend. Serve chilled, at room temperature, or stirred into hot dishes such as pasta or vegetables. Store in the refrigerator for up to 4 days.

Tomatoes

Tomato is one of the key components in Italian cooking, but other Mediterranean countries make liberal use of tomatoes, too. Fresh tomatoes taste fantastic, especially if you buy them vine ripened from a farmers' market or grow them yourself. For truly concentrated tomato flavor, however, sometimes I like to use dried tomatoes. They really give you the full impact of tomato flavor.

Pesto is a classic Italian pasta sauce made of basil, pine nuts, garlic, Parmesan cheese, and olive oil, but as long as we've got a green salsa, I want to include a red pesto. Pesto is supposed to have a big, bold flavor, and this red pesto fits that profile. Make sure you buy dried tomatoes that don't have additives. They are easy to dry yourself in a low oven overnight.

Red Pesto

Makes about 1 cup

This isn't technically a pesto, but you use it the same way. Instead of combining fresh basil with pine nuts, garlic, and olive oil (as in a regular pesto), this recipe uses sun-dried tomatoes pureed with olives, garlic, and olive oil. You still get a lot of taste in every spoonful of this piquant sauce, so toss just a little with a cup of hot cooked pasta, add a green salad, and you've got a fantastic and colorful light meal. You can also serve red pesto on meat or fish to jazz them up. This pesto should be thick but pourable. If it is too thick, add a little more olive oil.

10 sun-dried tomatoes, dry or oil-packed (rehydrate dried tomatoes in warm water for about 20 minutes, drain, and then use)

1 garlic clove, peeled

1/2 tablespoon crushed red pepper flakes

6 tablespoons extra-virgin olive oil (slightly less if using oil-packed tomatoes)

20 salt-cured olives, pitted

2 teaspoons chopped fresh thyme

1 tablespoon chopped fresh rosemary

1. Pulse all the ingredients in a food processor until well combined.

2. Store in the refrigerator for up to 2 weeks.

Good Taste
~ 47 ~

Balsamic Vinegar

Vinegar adds tang to many recipes, and a little goes a long way. Balsamic vinegar, however, is sweeter, more like syrup, and when it is of the highest quality, it is expensive. But many delicious and affordable balsamic vinegars are now available in the United States, and any of them will work in my recipes.

You may think of balsamic vinegar as an ingredient in salad dressing, since it is often used that way. However, in Italy, it is also a common foil for strawberries. In the Mediterranean, people eat fresh fruit when they want something sweet, and fruit is sometimes paired with cheese. In this recipe, try fruit, cheese, and balsamic syrup together to get a taste of what a real Mediterranean finish to a meal is all about.

Garden Strawberries

with Fresh Sheep's Cheese and Balsamic Syrup

Serves 4

Because of the time I spent at Old Chatham Sheepherding Company, I came to appreciate the full mellow flavor of sheep's cheese. I prefer it in this recipe, but you could also use fresh goat's milk or even a fresh soft cow's milk cheese. You can use a high-quality balsamic vinegar as is, without making the syrup.

½ pound fresh sheep's cheese   *1 quart strawberries*
Freshly ground black pepper to taste   *Balsamic Syrup (recipe follows)*

1. Scoop the cheese onto four plates.

2. Sprinkle each scoop of cheese with pepper.

3. Divide the strawberries between the four plates, arranging them around the cheese.

4. Drizzle the cheese and strawberries with balsamic syrup.

Balsamic Syrup

Makes about 1 cup

1 cup balsamic vinegar   *½ cup sugar*

1. Mix the vinegar and the sugar together in a small saucepan. Cook over high heat, stirring occasionally, until boiling.

2. Reduce the heat to medium and continue to cook until the mixture thickens to the consistency of syrup, stirring occasionally. This should take 10–15 minutes. Store in a glass jar for up to 1 month.

These are just a few of the tastes that distinguish and characterize Mediterranean food. I want you to try these things not so much to feel as if you are in the Mediterranean but to feel as if you can taste and appreciate anything. Remember that the key to eating in the style and spirit of the Mediterranean is to eat from a broad variety of fresh foods that come from the earth all around you or from the sea. To eat Mediterranean is to eat like a woman who appreciates life's great adventure, not like a woman who is too bored, busy, or distracted to savor the pleasures of the table.

This is just the beginning of your culinary journey and the transformation of your mind and body. Are your passions ignited yet? Are you getting excited about the food in your life and the life in your food? Have one more strawberry, and let's move on.

3

Abundant Variety

Mediterranean people eat an abundant variety of foods. Most Americans don't. The problem with eating a lot of the same thing is that you miss out on important nutrients that keep you strong, energized, and even better emotionally equipped to handle your life. Nutrient deficiencies can compromise a woman's immune system and can contribute to health problems down the line, not to mention low energy right now.

All the nutrients your body could ever need are available to you in abundance. They come from your mother, the Earth, and they are most potent in freshly picked seasonal fruits and vegetables. In the Mediterranean, plant foods really are the heart of the cuisine. Why do we tend to relegate just a little bit of our plates to fruits and vegetables, then overcook them or eat them when they are old or out of season? I'm sure I don't know! *C'est ridicule.*

But I do know that it's easy to get in a food rut. You find

something you like — Caesar salad, or pasta perhaps — and you stick with it. Maybe part of the problem is that even though Americans have access to foods from all over the planet, when your veggies are shipped from another country thousands of miles away, they just don't taste very good. Not only is this food far from being freshly picked (even if it is sold as "fresh" in the store), but to keep it from spoiling on its long journey, produce is often gassed to retard ripening, sprayed with pesticides to prevent infestation, and coated with wax to make it more durable. Does that sound tasty to you? Not to me, either.

Variety keeps your body and mind well nourished, your meals interesting, and even helps your body reach its ideal weight. Variety is incredibly important for weight loss. Think about what you tend to eat or binge on. Maybe it's chocolate or nachos or those salt-and-vinegar potato chips or even something seemingly innocuous such as protein shakes or one particular type of "diet" frozen dinner. Do you eat one thing almost every day? If so, that's too much. You're in a rut and your body is suffering.

Recent studies have linked high fruit and vegetable consumption with stronger bones (greater bone density) and a reduced risk for a number of common chronic diseases such as many types of cancer, diabetes, problems with skin and joints, cataracts, and even senility. For example, women who ate nine servings of fruits and vegetables per day for many years showed a 20 percent lower risk of coronary artery disease compared with women who ate just two and a half servings of fruits and vegetables each day. Because fruits and vegetables contain hundreds and maybe thousands of cancer-fighting phytochemicals, the more types you eat, the more phytochemical action you get. One of the most potent vegetables you can eat are calcium-rich dark leafy greens, a Mediterranean staple. I encourage you to enjoy them often, trying the many varieties, both raw and cooked.

Another interesting study looked specifically at variety in the diets of lean and obese people. Both had a varied diet, but the overweight people had a much greater variety of sweets, snacks, and high-density, high-calorie foods. The lean people ate a much greater variety of fruits and vegetables. Eating fruits and vegetables every single day really is the ultimate strategy for a woman's glowing health, long life, sharp mind, and slim, strong body.

In the Mediterranean, abundant fruit and vegetable variety is everywhere, but it is also local. You can't get every single fruit and vegetable on every day of the year when you live in Sicily or coastal Spain or Tunisia. Food comes into season on a rotating cycle according to when it grows, ripens, and is harvested. Some foods are preserved—salted and marinated in vinegar and oil or packed in dry salt—but these foods are used to enhance certain dishes and aren't the main focus of the meal. And even preserved locally grown food can be more nutritious than "fresh" food shipped from a continent away.

Eating seasonally brings the women and their families living in the Mediterranean into harmony with nature because what they take into themselves comes directly from the earth at that particular time. They don't fill up on preservatives, chemicals, processed food, old food . . . they eat what the earth offers during each season, when food tastes better and costs less.

American women and their families can eat like this, too. I do, and there is no reason you can't. Eating primarily fresh, seasonal food will give you new energy and a clean feeling. You'll begin to drop extra weight. You may even find that your thinking gets clearer and your outlook gets brighter.

> *The day is coming when a single carrot, freshly observed, will set off a revolution.*
> —**Paul Cézanne, French painter**

✳ A Closer Look at Variety

If you are reading this book, you may already be interested in eating fresher, better food and you may not eat a standard American diet, but let's think about that diet for a minute. Many American women eat only a handful of vegetables on a regular basis—tomatoes in the form of salsa and ketchup (one study I've seen listed ketchup as one of the major sources of vegetables in the American diet—I couldn't believe they considered it a vegetable!), along with potatoes (usually fried), lettuce (usually iceberg), carrots, and celery. American women also tend to eat a lot of processed food in the form of frozen, microwavable diet dinners that come with a side of vegetables. Those frozen dinners don't look very tasty to me.

With vegetables like these, it's no wonder that vegetables aren't the centerpiece of most American meals. In the Mediterranean, however, vegetables are stars. From tomatoes and eggplant, to peppers and olives, to garlic and onions, to leafy greens such as escarole, kale, Swiss chard, and spinach—each of these in a multitude of varieties, colors, sizes, textures, and shapes—vegetables are the heart of the meal. You'll even find fresh carrots, tasty potatoes, crisp celery, and Spanish salsa, but you would probably have a hard time finding ketchup. Then again, you'll never miss it. (And considering ketchup's high content of refined sugar—no wonder so many kids gobble it up—you are probably better off without it, anyway.)

If vegetables are the heart of Mediterranean cuisine, grains are the soul. Grains come in a similarly magnificent variety in the Mediterranean—farro, barley, wheat, semolina, and grain-like plant foods such as quinoa, amaranth, polenta, chickpeas, cannellini beans, black beans, and favas. Grains make up pilafs and cassoulets, add a depth of flavor and nutrient-dense fiber to soups, stews, and salads, and of course grains are what bread in all forms is all about.

What grains do most Americans eat? Packaged presliced bread, white rice, and lots of pasta. American women have so many grains available yet eat so few of them on a regular basis. Why eat spongy white bread in a bag and elbow macaroni when you can eat freshly baked sourdough bread, whole-grain pita bread, tabbouleh salad, couscous with savory vegetables and bits of chicken, polenta with homemade marinara sauce, or risotto with wild mushrooms?

And what about fruit? America's holy three—apples, bananas, and oranges—with the occasional handful of berries in a smoothie or cantaloupe or bunch of green grapes—seems meager against the huge variety of Mediterranean fruits: sweet wild strawberries and blueberries, tart blackberries and raspberries, luscious melons of all types, perfect peaches and plums, plump pears and apples, pomegranates and figs, and everything from nearby rather than shipped from faraway countries.

You can begin to take advantage of the immense variety around you by getting out of your personal rut. Identify the fruits, vegetables, and grains that you tend to eat out of habit, then look around you. What haven't you tried? What is available to you? This is one of the easiest and most enjoyable ways to begin nudging your diet toward a healthier and more Mediterranean style, to lose weight and feel better. How can you start adding more abundant variety to your diet?

> *Nothing great is produced suddenly, since not even the grape or the fig is. If you say to me now that you want a fig, I will answer to you that it requires time: let it flower first, then put forth fruit, and then ripen.*
>
> —**Epictetus, ancient Greek philosopher**

✳ Mediterranean Meal Making

To begin getting into the habit of eating Mediterranean style, let's practice Mediterranean meal making. These four simple meals use Mediterranean techniques and recipes, but you can incorporate the vegetables, fruits, breads, and grains that are freshest and seasonally available to you. This is what will make these meals truly Mediterranean in spirit.

Meal 1: Meze Plate

A wonderful way to experience more tastes in small amounts is to eat in the style of the meze platter. This concept is the same as tapas in Spain or antipasto in Italy—little tastes to share. In the Mediterranean, the meze plate is traditionally snack food served with drinks in the afternoon to fortify until dinner. Americans can enjoy these same foods in the form of a great, quick lunch. Share these little dishes with your family. One bruschetta, a scoop of tabbouleh salad, and two quarter pita wedges toasted—one spread with a dollop of hummus and the other with a spoonful of pepperonata—and you've got a healthy, low-fat, incredibly satisfying light meal or snack.

Fava and Pecorino Bruschetta

Serves 4 as part of a meze platter

This flavorful meze combines a crispy texture of toasted bread with tender fava beans and pecorino. You can double or triple this recipe for larger groups, or the recipe could serve two for lunch. Fava beans are popular in the Mediterranean, but they can be difficult to find in the United States. If you can't find them, you can substitute freshly picked peas, lima beans, or even green beans snapped into 1-inch pieces. If you want to try another cheese, look for a tangy sheep's cheese, or you can substitute a good Parmesan cheese.

4 baguette slices or other bread cut about ¼ inch thick

1 tablespoon plus one teaspoon extra-virgin olive oil

Salt and pepper to taste

1 garlic clove, peeled and halved

½ cup fava beans (or substitute lima beans, fresh peas, or green beans)

2 fresh mint leaves, roughly chopped

1 ounce fresh pecorino, sheep's cheese, or Parmesan cheese, shaved into shards with a vegetable peeler

1. Preheat the oven to 350°F. Brush the baguette slices on both sides with the tablespoon of olive oil, then season with salt and pepper. Bake the baguette slices on a baking sheet for 8–10 minutes, or until lightly golden. This turns them into crostini.

2. Rub the crostini with the garlic clove halves. Set aside.

3. Shuck the fava beans from the pods and immerse them in boiling salted water for about 2 minutes (put them in a colander to do this, so you can easily lift them back out). Rinse and peel the beans from their jackets.

4. Put the prepared fava beans in a bowl and drizzle with the remaining teaspoon of olive oil. Sprinkle with a little salt and pepper and the chopped mint. Mix thoroughly to combine.

5. Place a spoonful of the bean mixture onto each crostini and top with pecorino, sheep's cheese, or Parmesan and serve.

Pepperonata all'Abruzzese

Serves 4

This is pepperonata, or pepper relish, in the style of Abruzzo, a region east of Rome that often uses peppers in cooking. It is a fantastic meze to have around—it has hardly any fat or calories, but it is so full of flavor that you may never want to eat jarred salsa again. I like to keep this in a glass jar in the refrigerator for a snack. You can put the pepperonata on a crisp piece of toasted baguette or a toasted pita wedge, or you can just eat it with a spoon. It's that good. It also makes an excellent component of an antipasti platter, or it can be a topping for fish. To have more around, you can double this recipe.

Note: For the tomato puree, you can use a good-quality canned or jarred puree (I like Muir Glen), or just liquefy an extra tomato in a blender and freeze what you don't use, for future recipes.

3 tablespoons extra-virgin olive oil

1 medium red onion, peeled and coarsely chopped

2 red bell peppers, cored, seeded, and cut into ¼-inch strips

1 green bell pepper, cored, seeded, and cut into ¼-inch strips

1 jalapeño pepper, cored, seeded, and minced

1 red chile, such as Thai, cherry bomb, or pepperoncino, cored, seeded, and minced

3 whole peeled plum tomatoes with their juice, crushed (see below)

1 tablespoon chopped garlic

1 teaspoon ground cumin

1 teaspoon ground coriander

1 tablespoon tomato puree

1 tablespoon honey

2 tablespoons red wine vinegar

Salt and pepper to taste

Fresh oregano to taste

1. Heat two small sauté pans on the stove, one on medium heat with 1 tablespoon of the olive oil, the other on high heat with 2 tablespoons of the olive oil.

2. In the first pan over medium heat, cook the onions until they are moist and translucent, stirring occasionally.

3. In the second pan over high heat, sear the red and green bell peppers, jalapeño peppers, and red chiles, stirring constantly until softened.

4. When the peppers and chiles are cooked, add the tomatoes and toss for a minute, then remove this pan from the heat and set aside.

5. When the onions are soft, add the garlic and cook 2 more minutes. Then add the cumin and coriander, stirring to combine. Stir in the tomato puree and cook 4 more minutes. Add the honey and vinegar.

6. In a large bowl, combine the pepper mixture and the onion mixture, stirring until both mixtures are incorporated. Taste and add the salt, pepper, and oregano, according to what tastes good to you. Serve at room temperature as part of an antipasti platter or warm as a topping on fish. For variation, stir in chopped fresh basil just before serving.

• •

PEELING FRESH TOMATOES

To peel tomatoes: Using a slotted spoon, dunk the tomatoes into boiling water for about a minute, then dunk them in cold water. The skins should peel right off. In a pinch, you can use good-quality whole canned tomatoes, but when tomatoes are in season near you, there is no substitute for fresh.

• •

Hummus

With the increasing popularity of Middle Eastern restaurants, most Americans have at least heard of this protein-rich chickpea spread. Hummus is delicious "fast food" and you can even buy mixes in health food stores to make your own quickly ("just add water"), but this homemade version is almost as fast and the taste is much deeper and more interesting. In a pinch, you can substitute peanut butter or almond butter for the tahini. Use white pepper if you want a cleaner look for your hummus.

One 16-ounce can chickpeas (garbanzo beans), drained and rinsed

Freshly squeezed juice of 1 lemon

2 garlic cloves, peeled and minced (or use roasted garlic for a mellower flavor)

1/4 cup extra-virgin olive oil, plus more for garnish

2 tablespoons tahini (sesame paste)

1 tablespoon sesame seeds, plus more for garnish

Salt and pepper to taste

Chopped parsley for garnish

1. Puree all the ingredients except the garnishes in a food processor.

2. Heap the hummus in a serving bowl. Drizzle additional oil on top, then sprinkle with sesame seeds and chopped parsley.

Tzatziki

This fresh-tasting Greek salad combines cucumber with yogurt. Very simple, very delicious. I like to use sheep's yogurt for this recipe. You can skip the first step, salting the cucumbers, if you are pressed for time, but it really draws out the cucumber flavor while eliminating excess moisture and any bitterness from the seeds. If you think you don't like cucumbers, try this salting method and you might change your mind.

1 cucumber, peeled and diced
1 tablespoon salt, plus more to taste
2 cups plain yogurt
3 small garlic cloves, peeled and minced

1/4 teaspoon white pepper
1/2 teaspoon ground cumin
1/2 teaspoon ground coriander
3 tablespoons chopped fresh mint

1. Put the cucumbers in a colander and sprinkle with the tablespoon of salt. Let it sit and drain for 30 minutes.

2. In a medium bowl, combine the yogurt, garlic, white pepper, cumin, coriander, and chopped mint.

3. Stir in the salted cucumbers. Taste and add more salt if necessary. Serve at room temperature or chilled, as part of a meze platter.

Tabbouleh Salad

This salad is filling and nutritious but has very little fat. Cracked wheat is a high-fiber, high-nutrient whole grain that American women often overlook. It is a staple in the Eastern Mediterranean. This salad is great cold the next day for lunch and travels well, so you can take it to work with you.

1½ cups cracked wheat (tabbouleh or bulgur)

1½ cups warm water

1 bunch scallions, chopped

1 jalapeño pepper, cored and minced

3 tablespoons chopped fresh cilantro

3 tablespoons chopped fresh Italian parsley

2 garlic cloves, peeled and minced

1 medium red onion, peeled and minced

Freshly squeezed juice of 3 limes

¼ cup extra-virgin olive oil

Salt and pepper to taste

1 tablespoon green Tabasco, or more if needed

1 tablespoon fresh green coriander seeds, or ground coriander

½ teaspoon ground cumin

1. Place the cracked wheat in a large bowl, and pour the warm water entirely over it. Let sit for 20 minutes.

2. Meanwhile, place all the other ingredients in a mixing bowl, and mix well. Taste and adjust the seasonings, adding more salt, pepper, and Tabasco if necessary. Add this mixture to the cracked wheat and thoroughly combine. Serve at room temperature or chilled.

Meal 2: Soup and Salad Lunch

American women know all about the combination of soup and salad for lunch, but the soups and salads we choose to eat and to serve our families are surprisingly limited compared with the amazing variety in the Mediterranean. Soup and salad are ideal for featuring the freshest and most seasonally abundant produce. We serve several soups and salads at Primo. The selection constantly rotates according to what is coming out of the garden. A bowl of soup and a salad, each prepared with a Mediterranean flair and the freshest possible ingredients, make a perfect meal. Here is an example with two recipes that go well together.

A note about the rouille recipe that follows the soup recipe: This flavorful paste is great to keep in your refrigerator if you make soup frequently. Just stir it into broth-based soups to make them more exciting, using it as a condiment. It thickens your soup and adds an intense flavor that makes the soup more memorable and satisfying. You can also use it as a spread for crostini as part of an antipasto, or as a sauce for chicken or fish.

Bread and Fish Soup

This recipe is so filling and satisfying that you won't even notice how nutritious and low-fat it is. Using crusty or stale bread in the bottom of a soup bowl and drenching it in hot broth is a Mediterranean tradition that works with any soup from vegetable beef to minestrone. This is one of my favorites.

3 tablespoons extra-virgin olive oil

1 medium onion, peeled and roughly chopped

2 stalks celery, trimmed and roughly chopped

2 carrots, peeled and roughly chopped

1 large leek, white part diced and green part roughly chopped

3 garlic cloves, peeled and smashed

6 Roma tomatoes, cored and roughly chopped

1/2 teaspoon saffron threads (if you can't find saffron, use turmeric)

2 bay leaves

1 teaspoon crushed red pepper flakes

3 tablespoons tomato puree

2 cups dry white wine (Chardonnay or Chenin Blanc work well—avoid sweet wine)

1 1/2 quarts water

1 tablespoon unsalted butter

1 pound fish, such as whitefish, bass, halibut, or snapper, or a combination, cut into 1-inch cubes

4 tablespoons Rouille (recipe follows)

Salt and pepper to taste

2 cups torn pieces of crusty bread, toasted in the oven

1. In a stock pot, soup pot, or Dutch oven, heat the olive oil over medium heat. Add the onions, celery, carrots, and leek greens (not the white parts), and cook while stirring for 3–4 minutes.

2. Add the garlic and cook 3 more minutes. Add the tomatoes, saffron (crushing with the tips of your fingers), bay leaves, and red pepper flakes, and cook 2 minutes more. Add the tomato puree and cook 3–4 minutes. Add the wine. Stir well and cook

until the liquid mixture is reduced by half. This should take 20–30 minutes.

3. Add the water and bring to a boil. Reduce the heat and simmer 30 minutes. Cool slightly, then strain the soup stock through a mesh strainer, reserving the strained stock and discarding the vegetable parts.

4. In another large soup pot over medium-high heat, melt the butter and add the leek whites. Cook for 2 minutes, then add the cubed fish and the soup stock you just made, above. Bring to a boil, then reduce the heat to medium so it is simmering.

5. Swirl the rouille into the hot soup, then taste. Adjust the seasonings, adding salt and pepper if necessary. Remove the bay leaf.

6. To serve, place pieces of crusty bread in each of four serving bowls. Ladle the soup over the bread. You can garnish with fresh chopped oregano and parsley if you have them available.

Rouille

Makes 2 cups

A traditional French rouille isn't anything like this recipe — that cooked sauce thickener takes a long time and careful supervision to prepare. My rouille uses roasted peppers, bread crumbs, and olive oil for wonderful flavor and very little prep time.

You won't use all of this rouille in the recipe for Bread and Fish Soup, so save the rest to spice up other soups and stews or to use as a spread for bread or topping for fish or chicken. The peppers, garlic, and lemon combine to give a real Mediterranean flavor. The rouille should last for a week in the refrigerator.

2 roasted red bell peppers (see below)
1 jalapeño pepper, cored, seeded, and
   roughly chopped
6 garlic cloves, peeled

½ cup dried bread crumbs
½ cup extra-virgin olive oil
Freshly squeezed juice of 1 lemon
Salt and pepper to taste

1. Puree the roasted peppers, jalapeño peppers, garlic, and bread crumbs in a food processor.

2. With the processor running, slowly add the olive oil, then the lemon juice. Puree until smooth. Season with salt and pepper.

• •

ROASTING PEPPERS

Char peppers over an open flame, such as on a grill or under the broiler, until the skins are black, turning frequently. While they are hot, place them immediately in a bowl and cover it tightly with plastic wrap. Let them steam for about half an hour, then peel them. The skins should slide right off. Discard the skins, cores, and seeds. Try not to rinse them as you skin them; you want to retain the flavor.

• •

Lucy's Salad

We never remove Lucy's Salad from the menu at Primo. Yet it is among our most changeable items because it consists of whatever is very fresh, right now, today. Lucy is our gardener, and she knows what is exactly ready on any given day, so this salad always has a different character. You can do this, too. Use what comes right out of your garden or what you've just bought at the farmers' market.

8 cups fresh greens, types depending on the season:
- *Spring: spinach, sorrel, chives, chive blossoms, baby red oak leaf, wild dandelion, lovage*
- *Summer: baby romaine, nasturtium leaves and flowers, basil, amaranth, beet greens, arugula*
- *Fall/Winter: baby kale, wild mustard greens, lollo rosso, chicory, radicchio*

1 cup endive leaves
1 cup cherry tomatoes

Combine all the ingredients in a large salad bowl and toss thoroughly with your favorite dressing, such as a good red wine vinaigrette or a little olive oil, freshly squeezed lemon juice, salt, and pepper.

Meal 3: Vegetable Bounty

For good health, sometimes vegetables should be the star of a woman's meal. This simple menu combines vegetable-rich caponata with a salad of field greens and beets. Some high-flavor sheep's or goat's cheese adds protein, but the mosaic of colorful vegetables of different textures is what really makes the meal.

Caponata

This traditional Italian dish is a deliciously thick melding of eggplant and other summer vegetables with olive oil, garlic, balsamic vinegar, and tomato puree. The brown sugar gives it that characteristic jamlike consistency. Caponata is delicious smeared on thin slices of bread or crackers as part of an antipasti plate, or as a sandwich filling. You can scoop up the caponata with delicious crunchy endive leaves, which seem to be made for dipping, or spread it on the pita wedges or crusty bread you serve with the salad.

1/4 cup extra-virgin olive oil

2 garlic cloves, peeled and chopped

1 medium onion, peeled and diced small

1 large eggplant, peeled and diced small

1 red bell pepper, cored, seeded, and diced small

1 yellow bell pepper, cored, seeded, and diced small

1 medium zucchini, peeled and diced small

1/2 cup chopped fresh basil

1/2 cup balsamic vinegar

3 tablespoons brown sugar

2 tablespoons tomato puree

1/2 cup golden raisins, plumped in 2 tablespoons water or brandy for 20 minutes

1/2 cup diced celery, blanched in boiling water for 5 minutes

Salt and pepper to taste

1. In a medium sauté pan, heat the olive oil over high heat. Sauté the garlic and onions until the onions are translucent, about 5 minutes.

2. Add the eggplant, red peppers, and yellow peppers, and sauté until soft, about 5 more minutes. Add the zucchini and cook 2 more minutes.

3. Add the remaining ingredients and cook until the caponata thickens slightly, about 5 minutes. Taste and season with salt and pepper.

Field Greens with Roasted Beets

and Fresh Sheep's Cheese

Serves 4

This is a lovely salad to make in the spring when beets are at their peak and you can find really fresh field greens in the store, at the farmers' market, or from your own garden. If you can't find sheep's cheese, goat cheese works, too. Both kinds of cheese have a sharp note that plays nicely off the sweetness of the beets.

2 shallots, peeled and minced

1/4 cup red wine vinegar

1 tablespoon balsamic vinegar

Salt and pepper to taste

3/4 cup extra-virgin olive oil

4 fresh beets, any type

4 cups mesclun greens (field mix)

2 sprigs fresh basil (torn into bite-sized pieces)

2 sprigs fresh Italian parsley (pick the leaves from the stems)

1/2 bunch fresh chives, snipped into 1-inch lengths

2 heads Belgian endive

1/4 pound fresh sheep's cheese (or goat cheese)

1. First, make the vinaigrette. Place the shallots in a bowl and add the vinegars. Season with salt and pepper and let sit 15–20 minutes. Whisk in the olive oil and adjust the seasonings to taste. Set aside.

2. Prepare the beets. Preheat the oven to 400°F. Scrub the beets and wrap each one in foil. Roast for about 1 hour or until a knife slides in with ease. Set aside to cool. When cool, peel the beets and cut into wedges. Set aside.

3. In a large bowl, combine the mesclun greens, basil, parsley, and chives. Pour half the vinaigrette over the greens and toss until all the greens are coated.

4. To assemble the salads, arrange the endive on a platter or on four individual salad plates so that the leaves form a flower-petal pattern around the edge of the plate. Pile the salad greens in the middle. Arrange the beets on top of the salad greens and drizzle the beets with the remaining vinaigrette. Crumble the cheese over the top and sprinkle with freshly ground black pepper. You may serve it with crusty bread or pita wedges.

Meal 4: Simple But Elegant

Sometimes women really need to treat themselves to something elegant. This meal will let you do that without loading you down with a lot of fat, calories, and carbs.

Pissaladière

This Italian vegetable mix featuring tomatoes flavored with capers and anchovies is heaped into a prebaked tart shell. If you use individual tart shells, this also makes a beautiful hors d'oeuvre for company. For your simple but elegant lunch, serve pissaladière with a simple salad of fresh greens and your favorite vinaigrette.

1/4 cup extra-virgin olive oil

2 tablespoons chopped garlic

1 pound ripe tomatoes, skinned and chopped, or one 14-ounce can chopped tomatoes, with juice

2 tablespoons tomato puree

1 tablespoon chopped fresh oregano

1/2 teaspoon sugar

Salt and pepper to taste

3 tablespoons grated Parmesan cheese

2 tablespoons unsalted butter

3 medium onions, peeled and chopped

Crushed red pepper flakes to taste

1 tablespoon chopped capers with juice

2 fresh or canned anchovy fillets, rinsed, patted dry, and chopped

1 prebaked tart shell, puff pastry, or pizza dough shell

1 teaspoon chopped fresh thyme for garnish

1. In a medium sauté pan, heat the olive oil over medium heat. Add the garlic and cook until it is soft but not brown.

2. Add the tomatoes and tomato puree. Sprinkle with the oregano, sugar, salt, and pepper. Turn the heat to low and cook until the moisture has evaporated, about 15 minutes.

3. Mash up the tomatoes and stir in the cheese. Cook 2 more minutes, then remove from the heat and set aside to cool slightly.

4. Meanwhile, in a separate pan, heat the butter over medium heat and sauté the onions until they are translucent and soft, about 8 minutes. Add the crushed red pepper flakes, capers,

and anchovies, stirring to combine. Season with additional salt and pepper, and cool.

5. Preheat the oven to 350°F. Combine the tomato mixture with the onion mixture and stir until incorporated. Spoon into the prebaked tart shell and smooth the top. Bake until the vegetable mixture dries a little on top and sets, about 20 minutes.

6. Allow to cool slightly or to room temperature. You may wish to garnish with roasted peppers and olives and a sprinkle of thyme. Cut into wedges to serve.

Thoughts on Dessert

When you were a kid, your mom might have served dessert after dinner every night, and we do tend to crave something sweet at the end of the meal. Sweet tastes actually signal your body that the meal has come to an end and help you feel less hungry. But most adults can't get away with high-fat, high-sugar desserts every single day. These desserts are for very special occasions. For some simple and healthy desserts, see chapter 15.

In the Mediterranean, special desserts such as cakes and pastries are also reserved for special occasions, but people in the Mediterranean indulge daily in fresh fruit. Whatever fruit is ripest and seasonal makes an elegant end to your meal. You can eat fruit out of hand or prepare it in simple ways, such as fruit salad, poached pears and apples drizzled with a simple sweet sauce, or a platter of fresh-cut fruit and cheese for your family to share.

4

Why Olive Oil Is Not Fattening

To really embrace the Mediterranean way of eating, you must embrace olive oil. It's one of those basic ingredients essential to life in the Mediterranean and the main source of fat in the Mediterranean diet. For thousands of years, it has provided women living around the Mediterranean Sea with energy, flavor, and good health. Science now backs up those healthy benefits. A new study in 2005 shows that olive oil has antiinflammatory properties similar to pain relievers such as ibuprofen, offering beneficial effects for people with arthritis and other chronic pain. Olive oil may also protect against heart disease, stroke, and certain cancers.

Olive oil may be why women in the Mediterranean have incredibly low levels of heart disease and cancer. Olive oil contains primarily monounsaturated fats—the kind that increase your good cholesterol and decrease your bad cholesterol. Olive oil contains oleic acid, which has been shown to block some of the processes in the body linked to breast cancer. Olive oil also gives body and flavor to plant foods, so you don't feel deprived. People in the Mediterranean whisper about the secrets of olive oil for healthy hair, beautiful young skin, and well-lubricated joints. Studies may yet back up these claims, but just look at a gorgeous Greek woman with a celestial figure, or at Sophia Loren in all her Mediterranean agelessness, and ask yourself if olive oil isn't worth a try.

I think — and research supports this — that olive oil is crucial for weight loss and weight maintenance because of the satisfaction factor. A study of overweight men and women compared one group eating a low-fat diet with another eating a moderate-fat diet with the fat coming mostly from olive and canola oil, peanut butter, and nuts. Both groups had the same number of calories. Only 20 percent of the study participants in the low-fat group were able to stick to their diet, whereas over 50 percent of the moderate-fat group stuck to theirs. Participants who stayed with their diet lost about 11 pounds in one year, but the moderate-fat group kept the weight off. The researchers attributed the moderate-fat group's success to greater satisfaction with their food. The people in the moderate-fat group spontaneously increased their consumption of vegetables and fiber as well as protein. It seems including olive oil in the diet may even spawn additional healthy habits.

I find all this interesting, but what really intrigues me about olive oil is the taste. Olive oils aren't all the same. They come in a wide variety of styles, colors, and flavors, from rich, buttery Spanish olive oils to sharp, pungent, green Tuscan oils. Once almost exclusively the product of Italy, olive oil now comes from many different Mediterranean countries. California has a healthy olive oil industry, too. Besides Italy and Spain, other countries that produce good olive oils are Greece, France, Portugal, Turkey, Lebanon, Morocco, Syria, Tunisia, and beyond the Mediterranean, Australia, New Zealand, Chile, and Argentina. The two brands I use the most and recommend heartily for their wonderful flavors are Nuñez de Prado, my favorite 100 percent organic Spanish olive oil, and delicious Les Moulins Mahjoub from Tunisia, produced by the Mahjoub family. Both are fantastic.

I love to cook with olive oil because it makes food more satisfying and delicious, imparting that distinctive Mediterranean quality to food. You might be put off by the taste of a very strong olive oil the first time you try it, but many mild olive oils, particularly from Spain, have a beautiful and subtle flavor that adds just the right complexity to cooked foods and raw salads. Olive oil helps boost the natural flavor in food and makes you feel satiated without having to eat too much. That's where it can help you with your weight-loss goals.

The Mediterranean diet is *not* a low-fat diet, and olive oil is the one and only reason for this. Olive oil may be fat, but it doesn't make you fat. It actually makes you healthier, keeps your arteries clean, and contributes to a strong heart. I'm no doctor, but I've read many studies and accounts from health professionals that state in no uncertain terms why olive oil is better for your body than other types of fat, including butter and vegetable oils, which are primarily polyunsaturated fats. As so often happens, ancient wisdom emerges as very sensible in the modern world.

The whole Mediterranean, the sculpture, the palm, the gold beads, the bearded heroes, the wine, the ideas, the ships, the moonlight, the winged gorgons, the bronze men, the philosophers—all of it seems to rise in the sour, pungent taste of these black olives between the teeth. A taste older than meat, older than wine. A taste as old as cold water.

—Lawrence Durrell, novelist

☀ All About Olive Oil

If you browse the store shelves for olive oil, you will probably see a lot of choices. Because olive oil's health benefits have been so widely publicized, most grocery stores carry many different brands from different countries. But what's the difference, and how do you know which oils to choose?

Extra-virgin olive oil is the kind you have probably heard about the most. "Extra-virgin" refers to the level of oleic acid in the olive oil. The higher the level, the lower quality the oil. Extra-virgin olive oil has the lowest level, which must not exceed 0.8 percent. Back when olive oil was regularly pressed in big wooden presses, extra-virgin olive oil was from the first pressing. The oil from later pressings was of lesser quality. But now that most olive oil companies use more modern equipment, that definition no longer applies. Extra-virgin olive oil must be extracted through natural (mechanical but not chemical) means and is usually the most intensely flavored of all the olive oils.

Virgin olive oils are also extracted naturally, but those graded as "virgin" without the "extra" are those with an oleic acid content below 2 percent. They're better for cooking because they are less expensive and don't taste as interesting, whereas the pricier extra-virgin olive oil is best for eating raw, as in salad dressings or drizzled on vegetables, where you can really feature that olive oil flavor.

Other olive oils that aren't labeled "virgin" are chemically refined oils, so these processed products have a blander taste. They are sometimes called pure olive oil or refined olive oil.

Products labeled simply "olive oil" are usually a mix of refined oils and extra-virgin olive oils. A lot of the olive oil produced around the Mediterranean is of a low quality, so it has to be refined to make it suitable for human consumption. By the way, "first press" and "cold press" aren't official terms. Anyone can use them, so don't make these a reason to buy an oil. And don't be fooled by "light" or "lite" oil, either. All oil has the same amount of fat and calories. "Light" is an unregulated term, meaning the oil is light on flavor. In other words, tasteless. Because I am so committed to freshness and eating unprocessed food, I prefer to use extra-virgin oils that are not refined in my cooking.

And what about color? Color isn't always linked to taste, but it can be. Green oils are made from younger, less ripe olives. Yellow oils are made from more mature, ripe olives. Green oils sometimes have a sharp astringent taste, but sometimes they are very mellow. Some have a grassy bright flavor, and some will make your palate tingle. Yellow oils may look like melted butter, but some of these are also quite sharp. Others have a rich mellow flavor. The key to discovering which brands and flavors you like best—both for eating raw and for cooking—is in tasting.

☀ Tasting and Cooking with Olive Oil

Part of the joy of olive oil is its versatility. But you can't know how to use it well unless you learn how to taste it. You can start by browsing for olive oils in the store and noticing how different their colors appear. Prices vary, too, as olive oils can be quite expensive. Price isn't always indicative of quality. If you have the luxury of buying a few small bottles, you can taste them for yourself. Some gourmet food stores have samples they will let you taste, too.

Dip bits of French bread in each type, or taste with a spoon, and really notice the differences. Taste how some oils are harsh or tingly on your tongue. Some even feel prickly on your throat. (This is oleocanthal, the antiinflammatory substance in olive oil.) Some are rich and full, some light with barely any taste, some very reminiscent of olives, some less so. When you are cooking, you can think about what kind of tastes will match the foods you are preparing. For instance, mild oils are best when you want other subtle flavors to come through, as in a relish with roasted vegetables. Stronger oils balance zestier flavors or can be more interesting on salads.

> *Except the vine, there is no plant which bears a fruit of as great importance as the olive.*
> **— Pliny the Elder, ancient Roman philosopher**

Some women find the taste of olive oil too strong at first. If you don't care for the taste of a strong oil, don't just assume you don't like olive oil. Look for an oil with a mild or fruity flavor. Spanish oils tend to have a mild flavor compared with oils from Italy, so you might try one. The more you use olive oil, the more you are likely to begin to appreciate the unique flavor it imparts to food. You can even bake with mild oils instead of butter. Try my Olive Oil and Lemon–Scented Semolina Cake (page 303). Olive oil cakes and biscotti are favorites in Italy. Remember, the more you incorporate olive oil into your diet — the more olive oil becomes the principal source of fat in your diet — the more you will be eating in the real spirit of the Mediterranean.

✳ Nut Oils

Olive oil may be the principal source of fat in the Mediterranean diet, but it isn't the only oil. Many Mediterranean countries use nut oils to add flavor to salads, dressings, and antipasto platters, or even for frying, especially peanut oil (not really a nut oil, but it imparts a delicious, nutty flavor). Walnut oil, hazelnut oil, and sessame oil have a strong flavor indeed, so you need only a little bit. Try tasting a few of these oils, or mix a splash of nut oil into a basic vinaigrette and see what it does for salad greens. Of course, you can get the benefit of nut oils by eating nuts, too. Nuts are the perfect snack: convenient, fast, tasty, and filling. Plus, nuts are proven to be healthful and are a great tool to keep you on track in your quest for healthy eating. A 1992 study showed that study participants who ate nuts every day had a 60 percent lower rate of heart attacks than those who ate nuts less than once per month. Other studies since then have linked high nut consumption with lower risk of stroke, diabetes, and dementia. Eating nuts has even been linked to living longer.

The traditional American notion that nuts are fattening and therefore off-limits to dieters is quickly falling to the wayside as people get more interested in protein and seek out low-carb snacks. Nuts fit that dietary fad, but they are hardly faddish—they have been part of the human diet for thousands of years. And they don't make you fat, either. Like olive oil, nuts help you feel satisfied with less food. One study showed that regular nut eaters were actually thinner than people who rarely ate nuts. Another study compared two groups of dieters whose participants lost an average of 3 pounds over two weeks. One group ate pretzels before each meal; the other ate nuts. Even though the nuts had more calories and fat, researchers suspect both groups lost weight because the group eating nuts felt more satisfied and ate less food during the meal. Who knew delicious almonds, sweet cashews, crunchy walnuts, pistachios, and hazelnuts were "diet" foods?

✳ Incorporating Olive Oil into Your Diet

It's one thing to buy a bottle of olive oil and put it on the shelf in your pantry. But how do you use it? Try these delicious recipes that use olive oil as a primary ingredient. Making olive oil your principal source of fat really is simple. Just eat less meat, and when you cook with oil, use olive oil. If you can make these recipes a regular part of your diet, you will have made a big leap toward eating in the Mediterranean spirit. I bet you'll really begin to appreciate this versatile oil with the beautiful taste.

Bagna Cauda (Hot Bath)

Bagna cauda is a celebration dip that actually comes from northern Italy. It consists of warmed olive oil with garlic, anchovies, and just a spot of butter. The dip is put in a bowl over a flame and served with vegetables such as red pepper strips, cardoons (a winter root vegetable), celery, and endive. Even though bagna cauda is traditionally served at parties paired with red wine and not as a meal, I think it makes an excellent light lunch. I like to use whatever vegetables are seasonal and look fresh, so feel free to change the vegetables in this recipe depending on the time of year and what you can find. If you do decide to serve bagna cauda at a party, you can easily double the recipe.

VEGETABLES

4 cups mixed raw, roasted, or blanched
    seasonal vegetables
    Some options: baby carrots, baby
        beets, cardoons, onions,
        artichokes, broccoli, celery, bell
        peppers, mushrooms, summer
        squash, winter squash, endive

FOR THE HERB BRUSH

1 fresh sprig tarragon
1 fresh sprig rosemary
1 fresh sprig thyme
1 fresh sprig lavender

FOR THE BATH

1/2 cup extra-virgin olive oil
1 tablespoon unsalted butter
2 fresh or canned anchovy fillets,
    rinsed, patted dry, and minced
2 garlic cloves, peeled and minced

1. Arrange all the vegetables on a platter with a small bowl in the center or a preheated fondue pot.

2. Tie up all the herb sprigs by their stems with kitchen twine to make a brush.

Why Olive Oil Is Not Fattening

3. Combine the olive oil, butter, anchovies, and garlic in a saucepan and heat on medium until warm. Pour the warm oil into the bowl or fondue pot.

4. Dip the herb brush in the oil and brush it all over the vegetables. You can even dip the vegetables in the warm oil for extra flavor after using the herb brush.

Charred Squash Salad

Serves 4

This recipe makes a good summer lunch because it features those summer squash that are so ubiquitous. Too much zucchini in your garden? Use all zucchini. Or pick a colorful collection of squash from the farmers' market such as yellow squash, crookneck squash, and pattypan squash. This delicious salad is very easy. Pair it with a little pasta or bread, add some fish or a handful of nuts, and you've got a great meal.

Use plain olive oil instead of extra-virgin for charring the squash. Cooking at high temperatures compromises olive oil's flavor, so there isn't much point wasting the precious extra-virgin stuff for this step. Save it for the vinaigrette.

1 tablespoon virgin or refined olive oil

1 pound assorted summer squash (try zucchini, yellow squash, crookneck, or pattypan squash), cut into various shapes

1 pint cherry tomatoes

1 cup fresh chopped basil

1 small red onion, peeled and cut into strips

Salt and pepper to taste

Balsamic Vinaigrette (recipe follows)

1. Heat the olive oil in a cast iron pan until it is smoking hot. Add the squash and fry them quickly until they are charred. Remove from the heat and put the squash in a large bowl. Toss them with the tomatoes, basil, and red onions.

2. Season the vegetables with salt and pepper, then toss with the balsamic vinaigrette.

Balsamic Vinaigrette

Look for balsamic vinegar that comes from Italy. This versatile vinaigrette recipe is perfect with charred squash. You can also use it on salad greens.

1 shallot, peeled and minced

1½ tablespoons red wine vinegar

¼ cup balsamic vinegar

1 garlic clove, peeled and minced

½ cup virgin or refined olive oil

¼ cup extra-virgin olive oil

Salt and pepper to taste

1. Put the shallots in a bowl. Add the vinegars, and let stand for 15 minutes.

2. Stir in the garlic and oils, and season with salt and pepper.

Tortas

This beautifully festive recipe has several parts. You can make just the torta, or you can make as many of the accompanying condiments as you like. You can make it all ahead of time, too. Tortas are fun to make, packed into ring molds, then unmolded to reveal their attractive layers. Made with fresh vegetables that peak at the height of summer, flavorful olive oil, and tangy sheep's cheese (you can substitute goat cheese), a torta makes a complete lunch, especially when topped with tapenade (the recipe for tapenade is in chapter 2), hot pepper oil for extra intense flavor, and the flavorfully bitter watercress coulis as a sauce on the plate under the torta or drizzled on top. But these tortas taste perfectly good without adornment if you don't want to take the time to make the condiments. You don't need fancy ring molds to make this recipe, either. Just remove the tops and bottoms from six tuna cans and wash them thoroughly.

1 eggplant

1/2 cup virgin or refined olive oil

Salt and pepper to taste

1 medium zucchini, sliced thin
(a mandoline works well for this;
see page 103)

1 1/2 pounds fresh sheep's cheese

2 red bell peppers, charred, skinned,
seeded, and diced (see page 67)

1 tablespoon Tapenade (page 37),
optional

Red Pepper Oil (recipe follows) to
taste, optional

2 tablespoons Watercress Coulis
(recipe follows), optional

1. Preheat the oven to 350°F. Slice the eggplant into six 1-inch disk-shaped slices and brush each piece with olive oil, using about half the olive oil. Season with salt and pepper and place on a baking sheet. Bake the eggplant until it is soft, about 15 minutes. Set aside to cool.

2. Meanwhile, bring 2 quarts of salted water to a boil, and fill a large bowl with ice water. Add the zucchini to the boiling water and cook 1 minute. Remove the zucchini from the boiling water with a slotted spoon and put it into a wire strainer with a handle. Immediately plunge the zucchini into the ice water bath.

3. Assemble the torta: Place six ring molds (as described above) on a flat plate or cutting board. Place 1 slice of eggplant in each ring mold. Top each with a layer of sheep's cheese (I usually pipe this in using a pastry bag with a straight tip), then a layer of peppers. Top with another layer of cheese, then fan the zucchini slices on top so that they overlap each other.

4. Drizzle the tortas with the remaining olive oil and sprinkle with salt and pepper. Chill the tortas at least 1 hour. These can be made a day in advance.

5. To serve, unmold the tortas by carefully easing them out of the ring molds with a knife. If desired, top each torta with a spoonful of tapenade, drizzle with red pepper oil, and finish with a splash of watercress coulis. Serve with a green salad and crostini (see page 57).

Red Pepper Oil

This interesting and highly flavored spicy oil is a great condiment for vegetables, fish, or even bread. If you don't have a juicer, puree the peppers in a blender, then press through a strainer, reserving the juice. Squeeze out as much juice as you can and discard the pulp. This recipe makes 2 cups, so you will have plenty to drizzle on anything that needs a little extra zing. Keep it in a bottle in the refrigerator for up to a month, to use whenever you want to add some zing to your food.

3 red bell peppers, cored, seeded, and
    fed into a juice extractor
1 cup extra-virgin olive oil
Salt to taste

Cayenne pepper to taste
Freshly squeezed juice of 1 lemon, or
    to taste

1. Put the red pepper juice in a medium saucepan and heat on medium until the juice is reduced to a syrup, about 30 minutes. Cool.

2. Put the juice in a blender or food processor and blend slowly while adding the olive oil through the opening in the top.

3. Add the salt, cayenne pepper, and lemon juice and serve.

Watercress Coulis

Coulis are liquid vegetable, fruit, or fish purees you can stir into soups and stews for added flavor. This recipe features watercress and adds fresh flavor to vegetables and fish, or, as in this case, can be used as a sauce for tortas. You can also serve it as a chilled soup, and it tastes great with scallops or spooned over oysters and baked.

1 bunch watercress, stemmed	*1 small potato, peeled and sliced*
1 cup extra-virgin olive oil	*2 cups water*
1 medium onion, peeled and sliced	*Salt and pepper to taste*
1 garlic clove, peeled and minced	

1. Bring 2 quarts of salted water to a boil. Meanwhile, fill a large bowl with ice water.

2. Blanch the watercress in the boiling water for 2 minutes using a wire strainer with a handle, then plunge immediately into the ice water. Squeeze the excess water from the watercress. Set aside.

3. Heat 2 tablespoons of the olive oil in a sauté pan over medium heat. Add the onions and cook until translucent, about 10 minutes. Add the garlic and cook 2 more minutes.

4. Add the potatoes and water and bring to a boil. Reduce to a simmer and cook until the potatoes are soft, about 15 minutes.

5. Puree the reserved watercress and potato–onion mixture (including the cooking water) in a food processor, slowly drizzling in the remaining ¾ cup plus 2 tablespoons olive oil. Add salt and pepper to taste.

6. Strain the mixture through a mesh strainer and serve as a sauce.

Grilled Asparagus with Lemon

I love to grill vegetables. It really brings out their natural flavors. A little olive oil before grilling and a little more with fresh lemon juice as a dressing is all this tender vegetable needs. This recipe would also work with other grilling vegetables such as thick slices of zucchini or eggplant, bell pepper halves, or skewered mushrooms.

2 pounds fresh asparagus, stems
   trimmed
½ cup extra-virgin olive oil

Salt and pepper to taste
Freshly squeezed juice of 1 lemon

1. Preheat the grill to medium. Drizzle the asparagus with ¼ cup of the olive oil and season with salt and pepper.

2. Grill the asparagus on all sides over medium heat. Be careful not to overcook.

3. Arrange the asparagus on a platter and drizzle with the remaining ¼ cup olive oil and the lemon juice. Serve immediately.

✳ Olive Oil: The Mediterranean Diet Secret

Okay, so I'll say it one more time: The fat content of the Mediterranean diet works because most of it comes from olive oil and not from meat. The secret's out. Olive oil may be a fat, but it is *not* fattening. Eat less meat, and do what Sicilian grandmothers have done since they were little girls: drizzle wonderful olive oil over fresh baked bread instead of using butter. I once heard a Sicilian grandmother proclaim that eating olive oil "oils your insides." Maybe so . . . have you ever seen an old Sicilian face that wasn't beautiful?

5

To the Market and in the Garden

Chi cerca trova.
Who searches, finds.

I love to stroll through the gardens at Primo, choosing flowers for the tables or checking on the progress of the artichokes, cardoons, asparagus, tomatoes, and squash, or through the greenhouse where we grow exotic greens all winter long. To me, growing the food you will eat and serve to family and friends is such an important way to understand and be connected to the world around you. It makes eating a pursuit of pleasure and spirit, and it is very Mediterranean.

In the Mediterranean, food is such an integral part of life because people grow it themselves or know the people who grow it for them. Women choose their food with full attention, spending time in the marketplace carefully selecting the perfect vegetables and fruits worthy of their family table. They talk to the growers; they know the places the growers work and live. They buy food daily or a few times per week, so it is used at its peak. And they lovingly prepare this food and share it with their families.

When you connect with your food from its beginning—either growing it yourself and nurturing it to maturity or following the seasons and crop cycles with the growers at the farmers' market whose tables you patronize—you are more likely to pay attention to what you eat. Food becomes more than something you bought, unwrapped, and swallowed on your way from here to there. It becomes an event and a real celebration of life.

Involvement with your food and the knowledge of its origins is powerful. It connects you to your food in an organic and natural way. Not only does food taste better and fresher when it comes from nearby, but shopping, cooking, and eating with this connection to food from its beginning helps you to lose weight—that is, when you appreciate every bite, when each dish comes from somewhere familiar and holds all that meaning, mealtimes slow down and you get more from them. You savor the very best and reject anything less. You regain balance, and so does your body.

> *These are very nice ways to cook string beans, but they interfere with the poor vegetable's leading a life of its own.*
>
> **—Alice B. Toklas, American writer**

I'd like you to think about two things as you read this chapter: (1) whether you can do some of your own growing, even if you only have a tiny window box or a small space on a patio; (2) how you can take better advantage of local growers.

❋ You and a Garden

One of the reasons that Price and I knew the house and land in Maine were perfect for our restaurant was due to what we observed when we walked around the outdoor space. The acreage here at Primo is expansive and perfectly situated for a huge garden and two greenhouses. The garden is a constant adventure, always yielding new and beautiful things for us to serve in the restaurant. The food we serve is often quite literally just picked. You can't get fresher than that. We grow asparagus, fennel, shallots, garlic, endive, plum tomatoes, alpine strawberries, and squash, just to name a few of our crops. We also grow over two hundred varieties of flowers, both edible flowers for garnishing the plates at Primo and flowers for decorating the tables.

I love our tea garden, where we grow herbs for the teas and tisanes that we serve in the restaurant, and for our own personal use, too. (I told you that I drink herbal tea all day long.) Harvesting my own fresh herbs from the ground beneath my own feet means a lot to me. It connects me to this land, the town, and the climate. It makes me feel that I am a part of this place, and it gives me that Mediterranean sense of place, too. It's a wonderful feeling that Mediterranean women have enjoyed for centuries.

Our gardens are all organic. Our gardener, Lucy Yanz, tends to everything, nurturing vegetables and fruits that grow easily in Maine and many that wouldn't normally thrive in this colder coastal climate with its rocky soil, such as tomatoes, eggplant, cardoons, and artichokes. Lucy's crops thrive because of her care and skill, her natural methods, and her intuitive way of "listening" to the garden and understanding what the plants need.

Lucy says that what keeps her gardening is the trust that develops between herself and Nature through the process. She finds herself continually amazed at the way things grow and how gardens continue to change, evolve, and reinvent themselves with so little intervention. Lucy's one priority is to keep the soil healthy. She uses her intuition about what the plants need. Lucy spends a lot of time in the Primo gardens, observing and thinking and pondering. She is an excellent example of someone who lives a Mediterranean-spirited life, even though she is not of Mediterranean heritage. She works very hard, but she also understands that work is not about speed. It can be about slowing down, waking up, paying attention, and really being present with your work and yourself. When Lucy stands in the garden, she is really *in* the garden, and the garden speaks to her. Lucy's work becomes part of who she is, and who she is becomes a part of the earth she tends.

Lucy's approach to gardening is really very simple. Rather than focusing on what is wrong in the garden, she focuses on what is right. She works to keep the plants healthy because healthy plants tend to resist bugs and disease. She tries to understand just what the plants need at the most basic level, staying away from treating problems (unless they are crucial, and always organically) because Lucy believes quick fixes such as chemical sprays quickly become an addiction. Tuning in to what is really going on is time-consuming but more effective and natural. Lucy would rather step back and look at the big picture.

We have two greenhouses that provide us with greens year-round. One greenhouse is heated just above freezing to grow frost-hardy greens. The other is solar, and stays warm in winter purely by the heat of the sun—the greenhouse effect, working for us all through the Maine winter!

You don't need acreage to grow a garden. You don't even need a yard! If you have a yard, that's great. Dig a plot just large enough for what you are able to keep well watered, weeded, and tended. Grow some dependable vegetables for your area, but also experiment with a few that might be harder to grow. And don't get discouraged when things don't work. Nature is cyclical. You always have another growing season to try something new if you learn from your mistakes.

I hope you won't let lack of space dissuade you from plumbing the earth's bounty. For those who love to garden or love the idea, a backyard garden, whether extensive or small, can be a tremendously satisfying hobby. Maybe you would like to grow corn and beans, peas and lettuce, or big beefy tomatoes. Maybe a small herb garden appeals to you, or a tea garden like we have here at Primo. If you are lucky enough to have fruit trees, you probably already harvest some of your own produce, but you can also grow grape vines, plant a strawberry patch, or nurture blueberry, blackberry, raspberry, or even gooseberry bushes. You can grow vegetables and fruits in containers on a deck, or herb gardens in a sunny window.

Growing your own food adds a whole new dimension to understanding where your food comes from. You not only know your food's history, but you make it happen, nurturing the plants until they produce rewards. Gardening can become an almost spiritual pursuit if you let it, and there is no better way to eat your vegetables and fruits fresh.

> *I think this is what hooks one on gardening: it is the closest one can come to being present at the Creation.*
> — **Phyllis Theroux, American essayist**

Here are some tips from Lucy to help make your own home-gardening efforts a blossoming success:

1. Make compost. Composting is easy, even though some people have the impression it is difficult. Find a place in your yard for a pile. You can surround it with chicken wire or not. Compost all of your food scraps and mix them with your yard waste. Lucy says, "Most people have a pretty good balance on hand between their kitchen scraps and their yard waste, creating the perfect blend for compost." Turn it occasionally, mixing it up with a shovel. Water it occasionally, and voilà—black gold for your garden. Layer the compost over your garden whenever it is ready. "Compost is really the most natural process in the world. Nature does it all the time," says Lucy. You can even make small amounts of compost for container gardens in a bucket on your porch or deck. Alternate thin layers of grass clippings and dried leaves with food scraps. In just a few weeks, you'll have compost.

2. Prepare the soil. Lucy prefers not to disturb the natural soil layers by deep digging. Instead, she aerates the soil with a fork, then mixes compost into the first few inches of soil—the nutrients from the compost filter down into the soil around the roots of the plants, creating an instant and completely natural fertilizer. That's all Lucy uses. She also gives each plant the soil it needs. Any state agricultural extension will test your soil for a nominal fee, then tell you just what you need to add if you are growing organic vegetables (or anything else). When the soil is aerated, fed, and the right chemical composition, your plants will have the best possible chance at strength and health.

3. Don't get discouraged. Crop failure happens all the time, even to the most experienced gardeners. Just this year, Lucy lost a crop of artichokes. She says she put them out too soon. Artichokes are a hot-weather vegetable and they need to be managed just so. This year, it didn't work. But will Lucy quit? Certainly not. Lucy told me that if she had a graveyard for the plants she's killed over the years, it would take up the whole town of Rockland! "But failures are how you learn, not a reason to quit," says Lucy. "I know just how frustrating it can be when a plant or a row or the whole garden doesn't work the way you planned, and that can be compounded when you have a small garden. I garden for a living, so I have to keep going no matter what happens—no matter what has died or isn't coming on or gets eaten by bugs. I get very frustrated when I have to tell Melissa we don't have this or that because it all went bad at the same time, and I have to keep being positive, but when you are working in your own home garden and nobody is paying you to do it, you can get very frustrated."

Lucy believes that gardeners' failures are often due to poorly prepared soil and to planting too early. "Gardens tend to catch up if you plant them later than you think you can. You might feel like oh, it's too late, I didn't get my garden in on time, but try it. Better a little late than too early, and the garden will benefit from the longer days."

4. Be with your garden. "Slow down, be there, put aside what you've been told about gardening and just be there. There are so many books and opinions about gardening, but it is really something instinctual that most people already know how to do, even if they don't realize it," says Lucy. Spending time pulling weeds, assessing plant health, spreading compost, watering, harvesting, and observing all the garden's stages really puts you in touch with the Mediterranean way.

☀ Your Guide to Farmers' Markets

Much of what we don't grow on the land at Primo, I get from local growers right here in Rockland. So many local or regional farmers are producing gorgeous organic produce, artisanal cheeses, spices and herbs, nuts and seeds—and not just in Maine. Some of my favorites include York Hill Farm in New Sharon, Maine, for artisanal cheeses; Wild Asparagus Farm in Whitefield for Maine wildflower honey; Watershed Farm in Appleton, Maine, for organic vegetables; Peacemeal Farm in Dixmont, also for organic vegetables; Spear Farm in Warren for vegetables; and Anson Mills in Columbia, South Carolina, for organic grains like their fabulous polenta and wonderful farro. Chances are there are lots of local producers with fresh organic food right where you live.

Farmers' markets, natural food co-ops, and even roadside produce stands are great places to shop. Many areas have a community-supported agriculture (CSA) program. You sign up, then every week throughout the growing season, you get to pick up a big sack of fresh produce grown and freshly picked by the farmers in your own community. You'll get to eat seasonally the easy way, with all the very freshest and ripest produce handed to you. You'll eat more fruits and vegetables, you'll feel better, and you'll be connected to your community in a very meaningful way.

Browsing the farmers' market is fun, too. Visit with the growers and ask questions about the work they do, why they grow the crops they grow, how the weather is influencing this week's or month's or season's harvest. You never know what you might learn about why this batch of berries tastes better than the last, about the person who made the bread, or about why someone specializes in making a particular kind of cheese. Go to the farmers' market regularly so that the farmers and other artisanal producers get to know you. They might even start setting aside the best of what they've got just for you because they recognize that you truly appreciate the very best and freshest food. They also appreciate what *you* know. Tell them of things you remember from your childhood, a kind of special tomato or apple or bread, and see if they can help you find these items. Getting to know the people who grow the food you eat is a wonderful way to get more connected with your food and community.

Wouldn't you rather wander through the open air looking at freshly picked produce than push a cart through the fluorescent light of a megasupermarket? I know I would. Making weekly farmers' market visits a priority helps you schedule in some relaxing Mediterranean-style leisure time. It also gives you a great opportunity to get more variety in your diet. If you make it a point to try something new every time you visit the farmers' market, you will meet more people, try more things, train your palette to be even more discerning, and experience more of the adventure that eating should be.

I know this might sound like a lot of work, and it is surely faster to rush to the grocery store once a week, buy whatever you need, and be done with it. But taking the time to follow your food, choose it with care, and relish the sensual pleasures of touching and tasting as you decide what deserves to grace your dinner table—this embraces the spirit of eating in the Mediterranean.

Once you get home with your bundle of fresh food, the real fun starts: devising ways to serve this food in the tastiest ways possible. Sometimes, simple is best—thick, juicy slices of peaches or melons, tangy vine-ripened tomatoes topped with a sprinkle of salt and some fresh basil, salad greens just picked and drizzled with olive oil. But you can do a lot more with the fresh produce you find growing all around you. Here are some of my favorite recipes to inspire you.

• •

MANDOLINES

A mandoline is a French cooking tool that makes slicing vegetables and fruits practically effortless. Buy a good-quality mandoline—they can be pricey but will last for years with good care. I like the wonderful and versatile Bron-Coucke mandoline, which we use constantly in the restaurant. Just watch your fingers; the best mandolines are very sharp.

• •

Cherry Tomato Salad

This bright salad is perfect for using the fresh, colorful, small tomatoes you can often find in farmers' markets or that may overwhelm your garden come midsummer. Easy to make and delicious, this is a good lunch paired with some fresh cheese and bread. Or make crusty croutons and toss them right in the salad to make Panzanella, a Tuscan bread salad.

3 pints assorted small tomatoes (cherry, pear, grape, red, and yellow)
1 bunch of fresh basil
3 shallots, peeled and minced
1/4 cup balsamic vinegar
2 tablespoons red wine vinegar
1 tablespoon minced garlic
Salt and pepper to taste
3/4 cup extra-virgin olive oil

1. Cut the tomatoes in half and put them in a large bowl.

2. Chop the basil into very thin strips, called a chiffonade, and add to the tomatoes, and set aside.

3. Make the dressing. In a small bowl, combine the shallots, vinegars, garlic, salt, and pepper. Mix well, then let rest for 15 minutes.

4. Whisk the oil into the vinegar mixture a little at a time, then toss the dressing with the tomatoes and basil. Add more salt and pepper if needed. Chill until ready to serve.

Farmer's Omelet

Serves 2

Who says you can't eat vegetables for breakfast . . . or eggs for dinner? This quick meal is great for two people, for lunch or a light supper, especially if you can buy fresh eggs at your local market. The vegetables here are just suggestions. You can replace them with whatever is in season—tomatoes, avocados, asparagus, even winter greens lightly sautéed in a little olive oil before folding them into the eggs. Use your imagination with this versatile recipe.

1 tablespoon unsalted butter

1 leek, diced

5 eggs, beaten

3 red-skinned potatoes, quartered and boiled until tender

2 tablespoons fresh sheep's cheese

Salt and pepper to taste

1 tablespoon chopped fresh thyme

1. Heat a nonstick skillet over medium heat and add the butter. When the butter begins to foam, add the leeks and sauté for 2 minutes.

2. Add the eggs and scramble lightly with a rubber spatula until almost set. Smooth out an even layer.

3. Put the potatoes and sheep's cheese on one side of the omelet and fold the other side over as you ease the omelet onto a plate. Sprinkle with salt, pepper, and thyme. Share with someone you love.

Butternut Squash Soup

When fall begins, the farmers' markets fill up with apples and cider, winter squash and onions. This soup incorporates these delicious and warming fruits and vegetables, and it is something to look forward to all summer. If you want to make a lighter version, use milk or half-and-half instead of heavy cream. This recipe uses canola oil, which primarily contains monounsaturated fat such as olive oil but has an almost completely neutral taste, so it doesn't interfere with the taste of the squash and apples.

1 large butternut squash, halved lengthwise and seeded

1 tablespoon unsalted butter

1/4 cup canola oil

1 medium onion, peeled and coarsely chopped

1 tart apple such as Granny Smith, peeled and coarsely chopped

2 garlic cloves, peeled and minced

1 cup apple cider

1 quart chicken broth, vegetable stock, or water

2 cups water

1 bay leaf

Salt and pepper to taste

1 cup heavy cream, or use milk for a lighter soup

1/2 cup toasted pepitas (pumpkin seeds) for garnish

1. Preheat the oven to 400°F. Place the squash halves cut side down on a baking pan. Fill the pan with 1 inch of water. Roast in the oven until soft, 35–40 minutes, depending on the size of the squash. Scoop out the pulp into a bowl and set aside.

2. Heat the butter and canola oil in a stock pot. Add the onions and apples, and cook over medium heat until the onions are

translucent, about 5 minutes. Add the garlic, cook 2 more minutes, then add the squash pulp. Cook 5 minutes, stirring constantly.

3. Add the cider and continue cooking until the liquid is reduced by half, about 20 minutes. Add the chicken broth, 2 cups water, bay leaf, salt, and pepper. Bring the pot to a boil, then reduce the heat to medium-low and simmer 20 minutes.

4. Stir in the cream or milk, and cook 10 minutes. Remove from the heat and cool slightly. Puree with an immersion blender, or in a regular blender or food processor in small batches (be careful if the soup is still hot!). Taste and add more salt and pepper if necessary. Garnish with toasted pepitas.

5. Reheat until hot and serve with crostini and a green salad.

Green Tomato Marmalade

Makes 2 cups

Why make marmalade when you can buy grape jelly in the store? Because marmalade has chunks of real fruits including citrus peel, which is filled with nutrients, phytochemicals, and flavor. I love making unusual marmalades. This one is perfect when you've got lots of tomatoes on the way. The green tomatoes are a juicy, tart counterpoint to the citrus and sugar. This marmalade has so much flavor that just a little on your bread will keep you humming happily, especially if you know you or your local grower produced those lovely tomatoes.

Green tomato marmalade makes a great gift. You can also freeze this marmalade in small containers.

2 pounds green tomatoes, cored and chopped

1 organic orange, thinly sliced and seeded (leave the peel on)

1 organic lemon, thinly sliced and seeded (leave the peel on)

1½ cups sugar (or a little less)

¼ cup red wine vinegar (or a little less)

2 tablespoons fresh ginger root, peeled and finely chopped

½ teaspoon salt

½ teaspoon ground cloves

Pinch of cayenne pepper

1. Put all the ingredients in a covered pot and bring to a boil.

2. Uncover the pot and continue to boil the marmalade until the liquid is reduced enough to make it thick and syrupy, about 10 minutes. Stir often.

3. When the marmalade is the right consistency, remove from the heat and cool. Ladle into clean glass jars. This should keep in the refrigerator for about 1 week.

Vegetable Terrine

This beautiful vegetable terrine layers lots of fresh vegetables that you can find in the farmers' market or that you might grow yourself. Terrines are often made with layered meats or seafood, but this one is purely made with vegetables. It may sound complicated, but it's very fun to assemble.

Traditionally, terrines are served cold in slices, with tiny gherkin pickles and pickled onions. To make this one, use a terrine pan, which is like a long loaf pan with sides that come apart and a lid to press in the ingredients and compact them as they chill for easier slicing, or just use a loaf pan that you can cover with foil and weight down with another dish. This recipe makes a lot. The terrine is wonderful as a next-day leftover or as a party dish, or even put a slice on bread and enjoy as a sandwich.

3 large zucchini, peeled and thinly sliced lengthwise

3 long yellow squash, peeled and thinly sliced lengthwise

3 long eggplant, peeled and thinly sliced lengthwise

20 shiitake or crimini (baby bella) mushroom caps

1/2 cup extra-virgin olive oil

Crushed red pepper flakes to taste

Salt to taste

3 large red bell peppers

3 large yellow bell peppers

Pepper to taste

2 cups fresh spinach

10 thin leeks or shallots, white parts only, chopped

2 garlic cloves, peeled and minced

1. Preheat the oven to 400°F. Put the zucchini, squash, eggplant, and mushroom caps in a large roasting pan or cookie sheet. Brush them with olive oil and season with red pepper flakes and salt. Roast until tender, about 10 minutes.

2. Roast and peel the red and yellow bell peppers (see page 67), leaving them whole but pulling out the cores and seeds. Brush the roasted bell peppers with about 2 tablespoons olive oil, then season with red pepper flakes, salt, and pepper.

3. In a sauté pan, heat the remaining olive oil over medium-high heat and sauté the spinach with the leeks or shallots and garlic until the spinach is completely wilted. Squeeze dry between paper towels. Season with red pepper flakes, salt, and pepper.

4. Line the terrine mold with the sliced eggplant, overlapping layers until it is covered. Layer the remaining vegetables in the terrine: Begin with one layer of the squash strips, including zucchini, top with the mushrooms, peppers, and a thin layer of the spinach mixture. Repeat layers (it's okay if you run out of peppers and keep going with the other vegetables) until the mold is full. Put on the cover, or cover the loaf pan with foil and weight it down with another loaf pan and a brick or other weight. Press down.

5. Chill the terrine overnight, keeping the top weighted. To serve, remove the sides and slice, or just slice from the loaf pan and carefully remove.

Braised Romano Beans with Soffritto

Beans are another summer vegetable that can suddenly grow in abundance and leave you wondering what to do with them all. Or maybe the bright, crisp beans at the farmers' market are impossible to resist. Try this delicious recipe flavored with soffritto, an Italian mixture of onions, celery, and carrots gently sautéed in olive oil until soft.

2 tablespoons extra-virgin olive oil
1/2 cup Soffritto (recipe follows)
2 teaspoons minced garlic
2 teaspoons tomato puree
2 whole peeled tomatoes in their juice, crushed

1 sprig fresh rosemary
1 1/2 pounds Romano or other fresh green beans, trimmed
Salt and pepper to taste

1. Heat the olive oil in a sauté pan over medium heat. Add the soffritto and cook, stirring, for 3 minutes.

2. Add the garlic, tomato puree, and crushed tomatoes, stirring to combine. Add the rosemary sprig and beans, and toss to coat.

3. Add just enough water to cover the beans, and simmer until they are tender, 30–45 minutes. Remove the rosemary sprig before serving.

Soffritto

Makes about 5 cups

This recipe makes more soffritto than you will need for the Romano bean recipe. Keep the soffritto in a glass jar in the refrigerator for up to one week. Mix it into roasted peppers with some fresh herbs for a delicious antipasto.

2 cups chopped red onions
1 cup minced celery

1 cup chopped carrots or fennel
1 cup extra-virgin olive oil

Combine all the ingredients in a sauté pan over medium heat. Cook slowly for about 45 minutes, stirring occasionally, until the mixture is the color of straw.

If these recipes have inspired you to use fresh vegetables, don't stop here! Experiment with your own ideas. Tuck fresh steamed, sautéed, or roasted vegetables into omelets, sprinkle them on frittatas, roll them up in tortillas, pile them into sandwiches. Layer them, spice them, flavor them with herbs and citrus, put them into sauces, toss them into a stir-fry, or decorate your salad greens with them. Or just dip them, freshly picked, sun-ripe, and crisp, into a little bowl of olive oil. *Perfezione!*

6

Tapas Tastings:
COLOR, MORE FLAVOR, TEXTURE, AROMA

In the Mediterranean, food is an art form. Tapas, or the little dishes that keep women's stomachs happy until dinner, are like little sculptures. *Tapas* is the Spanish word for an assortment of little snacks, each with its own color, texture, and aroma. Traditionally served with sherry, beer, sangria, Cava, Txocali, wine, or other afternoon cocktails, tapas have recently become popular in the United States as people discover the thrill of getting to taste many delicious dishes without stuffing themselves. Instead of entrées, tapas restaurants offer a wide selection of tapas with which you can construct a meal of any size or character.

The tapas concept is a powerful one for weight loss, but it requires reorienting your thinking about meals just a little. We are conditioned to wait for the main course. No matter how much we nibble and snack our way up to it, we still think we have to eat the whole steak or chicken breast or slab of lasagna. With tapas, the nibbling and snacking *is* the main course. You might get a tiny plate of greens topped with marinated vegetables, a dish of chilled shrimp drizzled with a rich peanut sauce, a tabbouleh pilaf, and a plate of three amazing cheeses with a few baguette slices. Small bites, big flavor. Who needs a main course? That sounds like a meal to me.

☀ The Tapas Mentality

Adopting the tapas mentality can really help you when you are trying to plan meals or when you are simply rummaging through the refrigerator, looking for something to eat. Think: little tastes. It's a simple concept, but what it means for a woman trying to get her body to a healthy place is just this: *little* tastes. Take a few bites of this, a few bites of that. Notice each taste, move on to another, and when you've eaten a few good bites of a few good things, stop eating. You've had enough. You are supremely satisfied . . . as long as your brain isn't telling your stomach that it is waiting for the main course. What main course? Why a main course? Little tastes are much more exciting, surprising, mysterious even.

Eating this way is truly and essentially Mediterranean, not just Spanish. The idea of indulging in little tastes to fortify midday hunger is popular in many Mediterranean cultures. In Italy, the antipasto is a mosaic of beautiful foods for midday or preceding a meal. In France, the hors d'oeuvre not only precedes a meal but is meant to prepare all the senses by being visually lovely as well as delicious. In the eastern Mediterranean—Greece, Turkey, the Middle East, and North Africa—the meze platter serves a similar purpose to tapas—simple, satisfying snacks that sometime stand in for a more formal meal.

Just think about the possibilities for you. You can move

toward your ideal weight by indulging in little tastes of goat cheese, tangy ceviche, perfectly cooked mouthfuls of tender lamb, morsels of chicken tossed with juicy grapes and crunchy walnuts, a few spoonfuls of marinated white beans, a spicy tomato salsa on a piece of crispy bread, slices of Spanish sausage, roasted peppers stuffed with goat cheese and drizzled with olive oil—each little dish plays into the whole experience of taste and is a whole experience of its own, whispering of another land, of exotic cultures, but also of the passionate experience you have immediately as you taste.

IRENE'S STORY

Irene's father comes from Spain, and Irene grew up in southern California in the restaurant business. Her father's Spanish restaurant kept everyone in the family busy: cooking, hosting, waitressing, busing tables. The family always seemed to be eating, tasting, eating some more. Irene says that for Spaniards food means family, and that's just what the family restaurant was to her: "Unlike Americans these days, Spaniards believe food is to be savored, to be mulled over, never rushed, and never eaten alone."

In Spain and all around the Mediterranean, holidays, weekends, and special events are particularly centered around meals—lunch can often blend right into dinner. Irene remembers one holiday meal when the paella was done about 2:00 P.M.: "We ate, visited, ate, laughed, and talked and at about 5:00 P.M. the hat was being passed around for some money so someone could run to the store to buy fixings for dinner later that evening. But we never left the table and always had something to munch on before, during, and after the main meals."

When the restaurant closed and Irene turned from waitressing to more academic pursuits, she gained weight. "I think it had to do with the lack of daily exercise. Waitressing really kept me on my feet!" When she moved away from home for graduate school, not only was her life more sedentary, but she was thousands of miles away from her family and the big lively dinners she had grown up with. Life in grad school was much different than life in the restaurant business. Irene had to struggle with the loss of many aspects of the Mediterranean way of life—an active lifestyle, close proximity to family, access to the wide variety of high-quality plant foods grown locally. She experienced the struggle with weight so common to American women who sit at computers all day and don't have much time to eat well.

But Irene explains some things never fade from the consciousness of a woman raised in the Mediterranean spirit. "We always had balanced meals in my family: meat, vegetables, starches, and fruit for dessert. It was always good. Every so often we'd be treated to hot chocolate pudding over pieces of sourdough bread for breakfast. It tasted much better than it sounds! But this wasn't every day. This was special."

Irene still makes the food she eats special. Her new life as a professor at a small college in Virginia exists all the way across the continent from home, but some of her eating habits are still very close to home. No mediocre leftovers, no fast food—life is too short to eat anything of low quality! Even if she is the only one at the table, Irene cooks, sits down, and savors the experience. And when she cooks for her friends, everyone flocks to the table because her food is so memorable. Every little taste is an event, and in true Spanish style, Irene will raise her glass of Spanish tempranillo and make a toast: *Salud pesetas y amor y tiempo para gastarlas.* "Life, money, love, and the time to spend them." The Mediterranean diet may not be able to provide you with money or love, but it can certainly give you more energy for living and quite possibly a few more years of life. Here is Irene's family recipe, sent to us from her Spanish father, Frank Grau.

• •

Grau Family Paella Recipe

Serves 6 to 8

You can substitute different kinds of seafood or vegetables for those in this recipe, such as scallops for the clams and mussels, or add more shrimp or lobster instead of using crab legs. Use what is fresh and in season. You will need a 16- to 18-inch paella pan set over two burners for this recipe, or you can use two large cast iron skillets, dividing the paella between them. Or cut this recipe in half to serve three or four people, and use a 10- or 12-inch skillet. To serve this paella in true Grau-family fashion, set the paella pan or skillet on the table to serve, and let everyone eat from the side closest to where they sit. "The rule is that you eat only your 'slice,' and you don't pluck any seafood from anybody else's section," says Irene.

4 chicken legs

1½ pounds pork ribs or pork fillet

½ cup extra-virgin olive oil

1 tablespoon salt, plus additional to taste

12 large shrimp, peeled and deveined

8 mussels

1 small red bell pepper, cored, seeded, and cut into ¾-inch strips

1 small yellow bell pepper, cored, seeded, and cut into ¾-inch strips

1 small green bell pepper, cored, seeded, and cut into ¾-inch strips

1½ pounds green beans, trimmed

1 large tomato, cored and diced

1 medium onion, peeled and diced

4 garlic cloves, peeled and minced

2 cups long-grain rice

2 tablespoons paprika

6 cups water, fish stock, or chicken stock

1 pound king crab legs (precooked, available at most seafood counters)

4 littleneck clams (precooked, available at most seafood counters)

Pinch of saffron

1. Cut the chicken off the bone into chunks and cut the pork ribs into 3-inch lengths or the pork fillets into cubes.

2. Add the oil to the paella pan or skillets over medium heat, and add 1 tablespoon salt to the oil. When the oil is hot, add the chicken and pork, and cook until they just begin to brown, about 5 minutes.

3. Add the shrimp and mussels. Remove the shrimp as they turn pink and the mussels as they open, setting aside. Discard any mussels that do not open. Continue frying the chicken and pork until it is fully browned.

4. Add the bell peppers and green beans and cook for 2 minutes. Add the tomatoes, onions, and garlic and cook for 2 more minutes. Mix in the rice and add the paprika. Let the paella cook for 2 minutes longer.

5. Season the water or stock with the saffron and then add it to the pan. Distribute the rice evenly and then do not stir the rice again. Taste and season with more salt. Boil the paella until the stock is half absorbed.

6. Remove the top shells from the mussels and discard them. Discard any mussels that don't look good. Garnish the paella with the shrimp, clams, mussels, and crab, arranging everything so it is evenly distributed over the paella. Simmer until the rice is fully cooked and has a crust on the bottom.

✳ A Different Style of Eating

Tapas are simple to make and a pleasure to experience. They are also practical when you only have time to grab a quick bite. It might as well be a quick bite of something really fresh and good. Several small tapas dishes are usually a healthier, more varied, and less fat-laden option to a big restaurant meal. This is real food, not packaged snack food. This is snacking the Mediterranean way.

> *Fake food—I mean those patented substances chemically flavored and mechanically bulked out to kill the appetite and deceive the gut—is unnatural, almost immoral, a bane to good eating and good cooking.*
>
> **—Julia Child, chef**

Adjusting to a tapas style of eating makes a lot of sense. American women don't seem to have time to cook every day. But we do have a tendency to eat too much of one thing. With tapas, antipasti, hors d'oeuvre, and meze-style recipes, you get quick and simple food as well as a satisfying variety that keeps you perfectly happy with smaller portions. These little tastes indulge all the senses because they are fun to make, pretty to behold, and a delicious melding of textures in the mouth. In her classic cookbook from the 1970s written while pregnant with her son Carlo Jr., *In the Kitchen with Love*, Sophia Loren asserts that antipasti should be called "fun dishes" after the Italian word *sfizio*, which means "the urge to enjoy." She goes on to write, "Anything *sfizioso* whets the appetite, makes the mouth water, and rouses the spirit of the *bon vivant* who lives in the heart of all Italians."

Try any of these tapas-style recipes for a quick snack or light lunch. A collection of eight or nine dishes will serve a family of four for an easy supper. And don't limit yourself to the recipes in this chapter. Many other recipes throughout this book can be tapas. Keep them simple and keep portions to just a few bites.

Traditional Antipasto

In Italy, the antipasto platter is typically a selection of cold foods for snacking. You can use leftovers or put out purchased foods that are easy to find in any store. Mix fresh herbs into purchased products like marinated artichokes or red pepper strips to freshen the flavor. This makes a fun, quick lunch. Feel free to improvise, but here are some ingredients that would make up a traditional antipasto. You could also include other recipes from this chapter.

One 4-ounce jar high-quality marinated artichokes mixed with your own fresh, chopped herbs stirred in

1/2 cup roasted red pepper strips, homemade (see page 67) or jarred, sprinkled with a little red wine vinegar

1 cup assorted Mediterranean olives mixed with orange zest and fresh, chopped thyme

2 cups assorted raw vegetables such as celery, fennel, and radish

1 cup assorted roasted vegetables such as mushrooms, zucchini spears, and eggplant slices

4 ounces cubed lean ham, preferably prosciutto

4 ounces cubed mozzarella or sliced mozzarella di Bufala

4 ounces fresh sheep's milk or goat's milk cheese

1/2 cup vinaigrette for dipping

1/2 cup extra-virgin olive oil for dipping

1/2 cup hummus or white bean dip (homemade—page 61—or purchased)

8 toasted pita wedges or toasted baguette slices

Assemble all the ingredients on a large platter and serve cold.

Frico

Frico are crisp, lacy wafers traditionally made with Montasio cheese. Montasio is a cow's milk from Friuli–Venezia Giulia, adjacent to the Asiago cheese–producing area, where there is a pasture-terraced mountain called Montasio. It was awarded DOC (Denominazione de Origine Controllata) status in 1986. At that time, legal boundaries were established for the production of the cheese and the milk used to make it. It took the farmers thirty years to earn this valuable distinction. Montasio cheese is pressed, not heated or cooked. Aged from four months to two years, generally the product we see in the United States is about nine months old. You can substitute Asiago, Parmesan, or even Gruyère in this recipe. If you mix the cheese with the optional risotto, it makes a thicker crepe-like wafer with a creamy inside. This is a good way to use up leftover risotto (if your household ever experiences such a thing as leftover risotto!).

5 ounces Montasio cheese, grated on a   *1 ounce cooked risotto (optional)*
fine to medium grater

1. In a medium bowl, toss the cheese with the risotto, if using.

2. Heat a 7- or 8-inch nonstick skillet over medium heat. Sprinkle 1½ tablespoons of the cheese mixture into the pan to form a circle about 4 inches in diameter.

3. Cook until the cheese is melted. When it starts to bubble and turn golden, slide it out of the pan and onto a piece of paper towel to drain, patting both sides of any excess oil. Hold at room temperature on a cooling rack to keep the wafers crisp. You can rewarm them or serve at room temperature.

4. You can fill these wafers when warm, folding them over, or shape them into crisp baskets by pressing the warm wafers into greased muffin tins and letting them cool. Fill them at the last minute with ratatouille, caponata, fresh asparagus wrapped in prosciutto, a sausage and potato mixture, herbed goat cheese, or fresh greens such as arugula.

Alici Marinata

This unusual recipe is tastier than you might think if your only experience with anchovies is as an unappealing pizza topping. Serve on bruschetta—grilled or broiled bread brushed with olive oil—or on top of a green salad with some shaved fennel and olives.

½ cup red wine vinegar
1 garlic clove, peeled and cut into thin slivers
1 tablespoon chopped fresh herbs such as basil or tarragon

16 fresh good-quality Spanish "white" anchovy fillets
½ teaspoon sea salt
1 tablespoon extra-virgin olive oil
1 tablespoon chopped fresh oregano

1. Combine the vinegar, garlic, and herbs in a shallow glass baking pan.

2. Add the anchovy fillets, making sure they are coated in the marinade. Let them sit for 20 minutes. Shake the bowl or pan to make sure the vinegar is under the anchovy fillets.

3. Drain the anchovies. Add the sea salt, olive oil, and oregano, tossing to coat.

Ricotta-Stuffed Squash Blossoms

Serves 4

This beautiful dish uses the bright yellow flowers from your squash or zucchini plants. And yes, those are squash blossoms in the picture of me on the back of the jacket of this book. You can buy squash blossoms in farmers' markets or pick them out of your own garden. You won't need to let every flower turn into a zucchini, anyway—most gardeners get far more than they need. If you can't find sheep's ricotta, you can use regular ricotta made from cow's milk or goat's milk. If you can't find pecorino, use finely shaved Parmesan. You can serve these squash blossoms in several ways. They are good with the Charred Squash Salad (page 87) topped with Watercress Coulis (page 92) and Red Pepper Oil (page 91), or serve them as part of an antipasto or as a tapas dish along with sliced fresh tomatoes sprinkled with coarse sea salt and drizzled with balsamic vinaigrette.

8 squash blossoms

½ pound fresh sheep's ricotta, drained

2 egg yolks

Zest of 1 lemon

¼ cup grated pecorino cheese

Pinch of nutmeg

Salt and pepper to taste

1 tablespoon extra-virgin olive oil

1. Clean the squash blossoms by rinsing them lightly in cold water and checking to be sure they are free of bugs and foreign objects. Remove the center pistil out of each blossom by loosening it with your fingers and carefully pulling it out.

2. In a medium bowl, mix all the remaining ingredients except the olive oil and stir to combine. Taste and add more salt and pepper if necessary.

3. Preheat the oven to 350°F. Carefully stuff the squash flowers with the cheese mixture. You can do this with a spoon, but I prefer to use a pastry bag and pipe it in. Don't overfill the flowers. Pinch the ends closed.

4. Brush the stuffed flowers with the olive oil and sprinkle with a little more salt and pepper. Bake for 15 minutes, or until lightly brown. Serve warm.

White Bean Brandade

Serves 4

Technically, a brandade is a French dish made of pureed salt cod, but I like this version made with white beans. It is easier and very good for you, plus it has protein and fills you up without overloading you with salt and fat. Use it as a dip or as a side dish for grilled chicken or fish.

One 15-ounce can white beans
    (preferably cannellini), rinsed and
    drained
1½ cups extra-virgin olive oil
1 medium onion, peeled and diced
1 fennel bulb, diced
6 garlic cloves, peeled and minced

1 large red bell pepper, charred on an
    open flame, skinned, seeded, and
    diced (see page 67)
1 teaspoon red wine vinegar
Salt and pepper to taste
2 cups water or vegetable broth
2 tablespoons chopped fresh oregano

1. Divide the beans in half. Set aside.

2. In a large sauté pan, heat ½ cup of the olive oil over medium heat. Add the onions and fennel and cook until they are softened but not browned, 5–6 minutes. Add half of the garlic and cook 2 more minutes. Transfer to a bowl.

3. Add the red peppers, ½ cup of the remaining olive oil, and the vinegar to the bowl. Add half of the beans and toss well. Add salt and pepper. Set aside.

4. Puree the remaining beans with the remaining garlic in a food processor. Add salt and pepper to taste and the remaining ½ cup of oil. Add the water or vegetable broth a little at a time during the processing until a mashed potato–like consistency is reached.

5. Thoroughly combine the pureed beans with the unpureed bean–vegetable mixture. Garnish with oregano and serve at room temperature.

Tapas Tastings

Corn Relish

This recipe may sound more American than Mediterranean, but that's exactly the point—corn is available fresh in the United States in the summer, so making this relish is in the real spirit of the Mediterranean because you are preparing food that came right from where you live. Try it as part of an antipasto, or for lunch with a green salad topped with poached fish or chicken. This also makes a good picnic dish.

6 ears fresh corn on the cob, husks removed

1/4 cup plus 1 tablespoon extra-virgin olive oil

1 large red bell pepper, cored, seeded, and diced

1 large yellow bell pepper, cored, seeded, and diced

1 large green bell pepper, cored, seeded, and diced

1 medium red onion, peeled and diced

2 jalapeño peppers, seeded and minced (leave some seeds if you want the relish to be spicy)

1 tablespoon minced fresh sweet marjoram

1/4 cup freshly squeezed lime juice

Dash of green Tabasco sauce

Salt and pepper to taste

1. Using a sharp knife, cut the corn kernels off the cobs and put them in a bowl.

2. Heat 1 tablespoon of the olive oil in a large sauté pan over medium-high heat. Add the corn and cook 3–4 minutes until it brightens in color. Set aside in a bowl to cool.

3. In another bowl, combine the red, yellow, and green peppers, onions, jalapeños, and marjoram. Add the cooled corn, lime juice, Tabasco, remaining 1/4 cup olive oil, salt, and pepper. Stir well and serve at room temperature or chilled.

Prosciutto, Fennel, and Pear Salad

with Persimmon Vinaigrette

Serves 4

This elegant salad uses some classic Mediterranean tastes: prosciutto (Italian ham), fennel (with its taste of anise), fresh pears, and crisp greens. The vinaigrette is truly unique and this salad makes a light meal on its own, or serves as a beautiful component of an antipasto or as one of several small tapas dishes.

6 ounces prosciutto, sliced paper thin	1 Anjou pear (ripe but not mushy)
1 tablespoon extra-virgin olive oil	Persimmon Vinaigrette (recipe
6–8 cups crisp greens	follows)
½ bulb fennel, trimmed	Freshly ground black pepper to taste

1. Arrange the prosciutto in a ring around the outer rim of a platter. Cover with a moist paper towel if not using immediately.

2. When you are ready to assemble and serve the salad, drizzle the olive oil over the prosciutto. Set aside.

3. Put the greens in a large bowl. Shave the fennel very thin and toss with the greens. Peel and julienne the pear and toss with the greens.

4. Add the vinaigrette, tossing everything together well. Place the salad on the platter in the center of the prosciutto ring. Sprinkle with the pepper.

Persimmon Vinaigrette

This vinaigrette will keep in the refrigerator for about a week. If you can't find persimmons, use ripe plums.

2 small shallots, peeled and minced
¼ cup white wine vinegar
2 Hachiya persimmons (very ripe), or
   plums

¾ cup extra-virgin olive oil
Salt and pepper to taste

1. Put the shallots in a small bowl and cover with the vinegar. Set aside.

2. Cut each persimmon in half and discard the seeds. Scoop out all the pulp with a spoon. Coarsely chop the pulp and add it to the shallots and vinegar.

3. Whisk in the olive oil and season with salt and pepper.

Are you inspired to try some tapas creations of your own? A meal of tapas can be very easy. You don't even have to cook if you have fresh fruits, vegetables, beans, nuts, and cheese in your refrigerator. I'd like you to remember *little tastes*—*little*, because you don't need very much to get pleasure from your food; and *taste*, because if you don't sit down and pay attention to taste what you are eating, then you've just wasted an opportunity to indulge yourself in true Mediterranean fashion. Let yourself taste. Just a little. And reclaim the joy of eating again, without guilt, without regret. With unbridled passion.

7

Going Whole Grain

Pasta drenched in savory sauce, chewy, dense country bread drizzled in olive oil, creamy risotto studded with wild mushrooms, nutty brown rice, tender couscous . . . rich whole grains. Are they just a dream? No! They are the foundation of the Mediterranean diet. I'd be remiss not to throw in the terrific practical wisdom of Sophia Loren, our modern-day Mediterranean goddess, and I can imagine she said it with a characteristic flourish toward her own figure: "Everything you see here, I owe to spaghetti."

But you might be used to thinking you can't, or shouldn't, eat carbs. If you are lacking whole grains in your diet, you are missing a wonderful and versatile food group that should actually make up about half of what you consume each day. That doesn't mean you need to eat a mountain of pasta or a whole loaf of bread. Certainly not! You can bet Sophia Loren doesn't eat 2 or 3 cups of spaghetti at a time.

Pasta and bread are quintessential to Mediterranean life, but portions are restrained. A serving of pasta or rice is (brace yourself) actually only one-half cup cooked. A serving of bread? One thin slice, not two. And those giant puffy bagels you might be in the habit of eating for breakfast? A whole one is about three or four servings if you compare it to a small slice of bread.

Whole grains aren't the kind of carbs you may be used to eating. They are rich, nutty, nutrient-dense plant foods. In ancient cultures, they are *the* food. Whole grains are good for you, they fill you up, and they help you to stay slim and healthy.

The key to weight loss through whole grains is portion control. We are so used to eating more than just a half cup of pasta. You can make friends with carbs again by keeping your consumption in line with the actual amount your body needs and sticking mostly to whole grains such as brown rice, whole-wheat pasta, whole-grain bread, "old-fashioned" oatmeal, polenta, bulgur wheat, farro, buckwheat, amaranth, quinoa, and millet. In its revised food pyramid, the U.S. Department of Agriculture (USDA) lists grains as the category that should take up the greatest portion of your diet. The USDA recommends getting at least half your grains each day from whole-grain sources.

Noodles are not only amusing but delicious.
— **Julia Child, chef**

The problem with carbs most prevalent in the standard American diet is that most of them are refined. White bread, white pasta, white rice, instant oatmeal, cookies, snack cakes, candy bars . . . white flour and white sugar make up most of America's carbohydrate intake. In the Mediterranean, women eat carbs, but they probably wouldn't even grant that presliced squishy white stuff the noble title of "bread." Sure, we love our

Italian and French breads, which are often made with white flour, but they're also made with fermented sourdough and consumed in small amounts. Depending on the country, Mediterranean women also enjoy unprocessed whole grains in the forms of chewy country breads, homemade pastas, mouth-filling farro, rich polenta often topped with spicy sauce, chewy bulgur made into tabbouleh, and spicy couscous topped with exotically spiced vegetables.

Whole grains are more filling and better for your body than refined. They contain the carbohydrate-rich center as well as the nutrient-rich bran and germ. Whole grains contain vitamins, minerals, antioxidants, and other phytochemicals, which are substances in plants thought to have therapeutic effects, especially anticancer effects, even though they are not strictly nutrients.

One of the best things about whole grains is their rich fiber content. High-fiber diets have been linked to lower rates of many chronic diseases. Fiber reduces blood cholesterol levels, lowers the risk of heart disease, reduces blood pressure, stabilizes insulin levels, reduces the risk of some cancers (especially colon cancer), improves the function of the gastrointestinal tract, and has been associated with greater success at weight-control efforts.

Fiber comes in two types: soluble and insoluble. They are beneficial in different ways, although they both help fill you up so that you tend to eat less. The soluble kind comes in legumes such as soybeans and lentils, oatmeal, and many fruits and vegetables. Insoluble fiber is highly concentrated in wheat bran.

Fiber keeps the digestive tract running smoothly. Whole grains take longer to digest, so you don't get that spike in insulin levels that you get from refined grains and sugar. This spike is what makes you hungry again so quickly. It is this insulin spike that the low-carb craze tried to thwart, but you don't need to stuff yourself full of meat to do that job. You can keep your insulin levels nice and steady just by sticking to grains the way nature intended them: all in one piece.

Health benefits notwithstanding, whole grains taste better. They have a fuller, richer, nuttier taste that may surprise you if you are used to eating only refined grains. Whole grains are wonderful to cook with, and because they are so filling and complex in their flavor and texture, they really do work as the center of a meal. A Mediterranean meal often consists of small portions of whole grains topped with tiny bits of meat or fish in a sauce. What fills the rest of the plate? Fresh, bright, delicious greens and other vegetables, of course.

✴ Finding and Choosing Whole Grains

Whole grains are simply grains in their natural form, with the bran and germ intact. Refined grains have the bran and germ removed, leaving the carbohydrate-rich center of the grain. When you get rid of the bran, you also get rid of most of the grain's nutritional benefits: fiber, a rich source of B vitamins, minerals, and phytochemicals.

It isn't hard to find whole grains or to work them into your diet. Most grocery stores have whole-grain pasta, brown rice, and couscous. Many also include whole grains—sometimes in "instant" or easy-to-make versions—in the ethnic or health food sections of the store. Look for buckwheat as "kasha," bulgur as "tabbouleh," and pastas, baking mixes, and breads made with other grains such as spelt, amaranth, or quinoa. Food co-ops and health food stores are still more likely to stock some of the less common whole grains. Give them a try. They usually have more interesting and less processed foods, anyway.

When shopping for bread and pasta, look for labels such as "100% whole wheat." If the packaging says "whole wheat," that just means some of the flour is whole wheat but not all of it.

Here are some whole-grain descriptions so that you have an idea of what to buy. And don't forget—a single serving is just one-half cup. Enjoy every rich, nutty bite of these interesting grains.

Amaranth: This ancient "grain"—actually a plant—is related to the spinach plant and tastes a little like spinach. Many indigenous cultures use amaranth—the seeds, the leaves, and the flowers. Amaranth seeds are often used like grains—you can pop them like popcorn, grind them into flour for baking, or cook them like oatmeal. Amaranth is very nutritious and has high protein and fiber contents.

Barley: Barley is the most ancient cereal grain still used today. It has been traditionally used in bread and cereal preparations as well as for brewing beer. Up until the sixteenth century, barley was the grain most often used for bread making in Europe, until it was supplanted by wheat. It makes a sturdy, high-protein flatbread but also a nice porridge, and it's a good addition to vegetable soups and stews. You can also use it to make a pilaf, like rice. Barley was the grain originally used for polenta in Italy.

Buckwheat: Another ancient cereal, buckwheat has been used in Europe for centuries, cooked into a porridge, ground into flour to make crepes or pancakes, crushed and cooked into kasha (a Russian dish), or made into noodles, as it is in Japan. Kasha is available in many stores and is a quick and easy way to get buckwheat into your diet.

Bulgur: Bulgur is the Turkish name for a whole-wheat grain. To make bulgur, wheat is cooked, dried, and cracked. For meals, it is cooked again in an amount of cold water equal to the amount of bulgur until the water is absorbed, which usually takes about ten minutes. You can eat it in place of rice or potatoes. You can top it with stir-fried vegetables or chunky sauces. You can also stuff vegetables such as tomatoes or bell peppers with bulgur, or include it as a stuffing base for poultry instead of cubed bread. Mixed with tomatoes, fresh parsley, and vinaigrette dressing, it becomes tabbouleh salad.

Couscous: This North African "pasta" is made from hard-wheat semolina, the same stuff most pasta is made from. But couscous looks more like a grain because it is cut into very tiny pieces that are smaller than grains of rice. In Tunisia, it is sometimes made with green wheat. This staple of the eastern Mediterranean is cooked by covering it in steaming hot water and letting it absorb the water until it is al dente. Couscous is the national dish of three countries: Algeria, Morocco, and Tunisia. It is also a traditional dish in Sicily. It can be served with barbecued meat, cooked into spicy stew, or mixed with vegetables and chickpeas. You might mix it with fish and vegetables or with nuts and dried fruits. Serve it in pilaf form, or eat it like a hot cereal drizzled with honey, sprinkled with cinnamon, and softened with a little milk, or make it extra spicy with red peppers. Couscous is obviously versatile as well as easy to find and prepare.

Farro/Emmer Wheat/Spelt: Farro is an ancient variety of wheat that doesn't resemble the wheat we use today to make bread. It is very hard and must be soaked for a long time before cooking, after which it can be prepared like rice or used in soup or bread, as people like to do in Provence. Some people say farro and spelt are the same grain, but farro is actually the same as emmer wheat and spelt is a different cereal grain. Farro is commonly used in Tuscany in soups and salads.

Millet: Millet is a grain that grows well in dry soil and has been served for thousands of years in Italy, Africa, and Asia. It is often used to make flour and is also used for poultry feed. The birdseed you use in your outdoor feeders probably contains a lot of millet, but millet isn't just for the birds. Cook it as a hot cereal or side dish just like you would cook bulgur: in an amount of water equal to the amount of millet, boil it for about ten minutes or until all the water is absorbed. Try it with a spicy or tangy sauce, as you might with rice or polenta.

Oats: You know it as oatmeal, but try the steel-cut kind for a chewier, nuttier, more whole-grain cereal experience. Or grind up old-fashioned oats in the blender and use the flour in baking. Oats are a great source of soluble fiber. Oats are more traditional for northern Europe and Great Britain, but they are widely available in the United States and so nutritious that they are worth including in a Mediterranean diet plan.

Polenta: Polenta is just porridge made from coarsely ground cornmeal. You can eat it like porridge (cook it like oatmeal), or you can let the porridge chill and slice it into blocks, then fry it briefly in a little olive oil and douse it in a chunky tomato sauce. *Very* Italian. It also makes a delicious breakfast topped with scrambled eggs, onions, bell peppers, and tomatoes.

Quinoa: Also not technically a grain but used like one, quinoa is actually a seed from a South American plant. It can be cooked as a grain like rice or ground into flour for baking. You can sometimes find breakfast cereals, baked goods, or pastas made with quinoa.

✳ What About Bread?

When it comes to bread, you can eat it! Yes, you can! But forget about the white, packaged, presliced stuff that you can roll into a tight little ball. Do you think people in Sicily would eat that kind of processed nonsense? Never! Choose bread that is dense, chewy, and grainy. Try rye breads, rustic whole-wheat country breads, flatbreads, and sourdough levain.

We are lucky here at Primo because Price bakes such fantastic and memorable breads, but don't feel bad if you're not up to the task of making your own. Most people in the Mediterranean don't! Instead, people typically visit the neighborhood bakery each day for fresh bread and carry it home under their arms (or in their bicycle baskets). Because there are so many grocery stores and bakeries in the United States, you can do the same. Bread baking is a sort of meditative act, however, and good exercise, too. It isn't hard, but it does take time because the dough must be mixed, then set aside to rise, then mixed again, then set aside to rise again. This kind of slow, careful, attentive preparation is certainly in the spirit of eating in the Mediterranean style.

If you have a day at home, you might want to try baking bread. Otherwise, be choosy about your bread. Pick the freshest, the best, the whole-grain and sourdough options, and eat just enough to really please you. Use leftovers for bread crumbs, crostini, or croutons. No need to overdo it—just have the slice you want and savor it. Then move on to the next course.

To get you started, try Price's recipe for this simple whole-grain flatbread.

Piadina

This Italian flatbread is flexible enough that you can add your own fresh herbs, grated cheese, chopped greens, or whatever you like. Price's recipe incorporates buckwheat, whole-wheat, graham, and bread flour for a delicious whole-grain treat that is super quick to prepare. Use it as part of an antipasto or put some grilled vegetables and cheese on top for a delicious lunch.

1/4 cup buckwheat flour
1/4 cup whole-wheat flour
1/4 cup graham flour
1 1/2 cups bread flour, plus a few
   handfuls more for rolling out
2 teaspoons sea salt, plus more for
   garnish

1 teaspoon baking powder
1/4 cup extra-virgin olive oil, plus more
   for garnish
1 1/4 cups warm whole milk

1. Put all the dry ingredients into a large bowl. Add the olive oil and milk and mix with a wooden spoon until the mixture forms a dough, adding more flour if it is too sticky. Cover with a tea towel and let the dough rest for 10 minutes.

2. Shape the dough into 4-ounce balls and set them on a tray or towel. Let them rest for 10 minutes. Meanwhile, preheat a grill or pancake griddle (you can also use a large sauté pan) over medium-high heat.

3. Roll out each piece of dough on a floured surface until it is about 12 inches in diameter. It doesn't have to be a perfect circle. Place the rolled-out piadina, one at a time, on the grill or griddle and cook for 1–2 minutes on each side.

4. Brush with olive oil, sprinkle with sea salt, and serve warm.

✳ Cooking with Whole Grains

I love to cook with whole grains, and Price loves baking with them. They really are at the center of Mediterranean eating, and they are so versatile that you can shape them in many ways by adding different spices, herbs, cheeses, and oils, not to mention the various things you can put on them, from the curried couscous to the farro ragout recipes that follow. Whole grains can make you feel very good. Here are some of my favorite recipes to get you started experimenting in the world of Mediterranean grains.

Farro Salad Agrodolce

Farro is such an overlooked grain, and so delicious, especially the farro produced by Anson Mills. This salad has the classic Mediterranean sweet-and-sour flavor called *agrodolce*. It is wonderful served at room temperature with hot dishes like lamb or grilled fish, or served cold as part of an antipasto. I often eat a bowl of this for lunch.

½ pound dry farro, preferably Anson Mills

½ cup lightly toasted pine nuts (toast in a cast iron skillet on medium for about 2 minutes)

1 bunch (about 5) chopped scallions, white and some of the green parts

½ cup golden raisins, plumped for 15 minutes in ¼ cup sherry vinegar then drained

1 tablespoon chopped fresh thyme

¼ cup extra-virgin olive oil

Salt and pepper to taste

1. Cover the farro with cold water in a saucepan and bring it to a boil over high heat. When it boils, remove it from the heat and strain off the cooking liquid. Repeat this process again with more water, but when the farro comes to a boil, lower the heat to medium and simmer until the farro is tender, about 10 minutes. Drain the farro.

2. Add the pine nuts, scallions, plumped raisins, thyme, olive oil, salt, and pepper. Serve at room temperature or chilled.

Curried Couscous Pilaf

SERVES 4

This twist on plain couscous adds spice, color, and texture to chicken, fish, or tofu. Or enjoy this dish as a simple salad for lunch.

1 cup couscous (the larger-grained variety, if you can find it, but any type will work)
1/4 cup Curry Oil (recipe follows)
1 cup boiling water
1/2 cup dried currants, plumped in 3 tablespoons hot water
1/2 bunch scallions
1 fresh jalapeño pepper, seeded and diced very small
1 carrot, peeled and diced very small
1/2 red bell pepper, cored, seeded, and diced very small
1/2 red onion, peeled and diced very small
Salt and pepper to taste
Green Tabasco sauce to taste
1 tablespoon freshly squeezed lime juice
1 1/2 teaspoons chopped fresh mint
1 1/2 teaspoons chopped fresh cilantro

1. Mix the couscous with the curry oil in a stainless steel bowl. Pour the boiling water over the couscous mixture. Cover the bowl with plastic wrap and set aside.

3. Mix the currants, scallions, jalapeños, carrots, red peppers, and onions into the couscous. Season with salt and pepper, green Tabasco, and the lime juice.

4. Garnish with the chopped mint and cilantro. Serve at room temperature.

Curry Oil

Makes about 1 cup

This curry oil is good for drizzling over any cooked whole grains, from brown rice to farro to couscous. It's also good on fish or pasta. You need only a little. Curry oil will keep up to a month in a glass jar in the refrigerator.

¼ cup spicy curry powder　　　　　　*1 cup virgin olive oil*
1 teaspoon to 1 tablespoon water

1. Moisten the curry powder with enough water to make a paste. Whisk in the olive oil.

2. Let the curry oil steep overnight, mixing occasionally.

3. Before straining, make sure the curry powder has settled to the bottom and do not mix. Strain through a fine mesh strainer without pouring the curry powder through. You can reuse the paste to make a second batch of oil.

Creamy Polenta

This is true comfort food with just a hint of spiciness from the green Tabasco sauce. Polenta is versatile. It goes well with just about any meat, poultry, or seafood. It also makes a great base for interesting additions. You can add mashed sweet potatoes, sautéed corn and peppers, roasted garlic, Parmesan cheese, herbs—anything you want. Try stirring in Wilted Swiss Chard (page 194), Toscano kale, or collard greens. Let your creative Mediterranean spirit loose! I just love Anson Mills polenta and always use it for this recipe.

2 cups milk, plus more if needed

½ teaspoon minced garlic

⅔ cup quick-cooking polenta (you can also use stone-ground cornmeal)

1 tablespoon unsalted butter

Salt and pepper to taste

Green Tabasco sauce to taste

1. Combine the milk and garlic in a medium saucepan over high heat and bring almost to a boil. Watch carefully so that the milk doesn't boil over.

2. Slowly add the polenta, stirring continually, and cook for 6–8 minutes, or until it thickens to a porridge consistency.

3. Swirl in the butter. Add the salt, pepper, and Tabasco. Adjust the consistency if necessary with more milk. Stir in other additions if you wish, then remove from the heat and keep warm until serving.

Tuscan Bread Salad

Serves 4

I like to make this bread salad with levain, which is a type of sourdough using wild yeasts and rye flour, but you can use any rustic country bread. Avoid soft bread that will turn to mush when touched by dressing.

½ loaf levain sourdough, crust
   removed, torn into chunks
¾ cup plus 1 tablespoon extra-virgin
   olive oil
Salt and pepper to taste
2 shallots, peeled and minced
½ cup white wine vinegar

1 tablespoon whole-grain mustard
1 teaspoon Dijon mustard
2 bunches arugula
½ cup pine nuts
½ cup dried currants, plumped in 2
   tablespoons warm water for about
   10 minutes

1. Preheat the oven to 400°F. Put the bread chunks in a bowl and toss with 1 tablespoon olive oil and a little salt and pepper. Spread the bread chunks on a baking sheet and toast until light golden brown, about 15 minutes. Set aside.

2. Place the shallots in a bowl and add the vinegar and mustards. Let this mixture steep for at least 10 minutes.

3. Whisk the remaining ¾ cup oil into the shallot mixture, and add salt and pepper.

4. Place the arugula in a bowl with the bread, pine nuts, and currants. Toss with the vinaigrette and serve.

Wild Mushroom Risotto

Risotto is the ultimate comfort food, and this version is always popular. Flavored with rich, earthy wild mushrooms set against creamy, savory, tender rice, this so-called side dish might just eclipse anything you choose to call a main course.

3½ cups chicken or vegetable stock or broth (or water)

2 tablespoons unsalted butter

2 tablespoons extra-virgin olive oil

½ onion, finely chopped

1 cup assorted wild mushrooms (try chanterelle, black trumpet, porcini, portobello, shiitake, or domestic mushrooms—soak any dried mushrooms in hot water for 15 minutes to rehydrate before using)

1 tablespoon minced garlic

1 cup Arborio rice

1 bay leaf

¼ cup dry white wine

½ cup finely grated Parmesan cheese

Salt and pepper to taste

1. Put the stock in a large saucepan and heat on medium. Bring it to a simmer and keep it simmering.

2. In a separate large saucepan or Dutch oven over medium heat, add 1 tablespoon of the butter and the olive oil. Add the onions and stir, sautéing until translucent, about 8 minutes. Add the mushrooms and cook, stirring, until their juices evaporate, about 5 minutes. Add the garlic and cook 2 more minutes.

3. Add the rice and cook until it is coated with the oil, stirring constantly. Add the bay leaf and wine. Cook until all the wine has evaporated, about 10 minutes.

4. Add the warm stock ½ cup at a time, stirring constantly until it is absorbed. Continue this process until all the stock is gone, adding just a little at a time and letting it slowly infuse the risotto. This should take about 30 minutes or so.

5. Remove the risotto from the heat and add the remaining 1 tablespoon butter and the Parmesan. Taste and add salt and pepper. Remove the bay leaf and serve immediately.

Farro Ragout

Spoon this delicious vegetable ragout onto a plate and pile briefly sautéed dark bitter greens (spinach, kale, collard greens, or Swiss chard) in the center. Top with 3 ounces of broiled fish or chicken if you wish. The farro and chestnut combination makes this dish "meaty" enough on its own.

1 tablespoon extra-virgin olive oil

1½ cups peeled, seeded, and diced butternut squash

Salt and pepper to taste

1 teaspoon chopped garlic

½ cup good-quality farro, preferably Anson Mills, cooked according to package directions

½ cup roasted, peeled, and chopped chestnuts (purchase roasted chestnuts, or roast and peel them yourself on a grill or in a 425°F oven for 10–20 minutes; cut a slit in each chestnut before roasting to prevent them from bursting)

½ cup chicken or vegetable stock or broth

1. Heat an ovenproof large skillet over medium-high heat and add the olive oil. When the olive oil begins to smoke, add the squash, salt, and pepper. Don't move the pan or the squash until the squash starts to brown, then toss or stir it until it has browned on all sides, about 5 minutes.

2. Reduce the heat to medium, add the garlic, and cook 2 minutes. Add the farro, chestnuts, and stock. Bring to a boil and boil for 2 minutes, stirring occasionally. Adjust the seasonings. Serve hot or warm.

I hope you are inspired to try some whole grains you've never tried before and to eat more of those you already know you like. If you think brown rice, oatmeal, or other whole grains are dull, reconsider them through the lens of these recipes. Whole grains highlight the flavors of vegetables, fruits, spices, olive oil, meat, and fish. They're too nutritionally important to pass up, too filling to avoid if you are trying to lose weight, and too delicious to miss out on if you really want to embrace the Mediterranean way of eating.

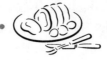

8

Madonna of Moderation

Meglio un uovo oggi che una gallina domani.
Better an egg today than a chicken tomorrow.

Being a butcher, my grandfather Primo used to bring home varieties and cuts of meat that most of my friends had never heard of. We didn't just eat steak and chicken. We ate duck, rabbit, and guinea hen. We had cuts of meat you never see in restaurants. But even with all this carnivorous bounty, our family didn't focus on the meat. We ate in the Mediterranean style, where meat was a special treat and the feature of a meal maybe once each week. Otherwise, meat, poultry, fish, eggs, and other high-protein foods were flavoring components of a meal, not the centerpiece.

This is the way meat is typically used in Mediterranean cuisine—as a flavoring in sauces, stews, or mixed in with vegetables and grains. Rarely is a hunk of meat the primary component in the meal. In the traditional Mediterranean, eating like this would be too costly. While people living in the Mediterranean in the 1950s often cited meat as the one food ingredient they would have *liked* more often, the reality for them was that meat was a luxury and an indulgence for special occasions.

In the United States, however, we have an abundance of meat and can usually purchase, prepare, and eat it whenever we want to. But this doesn't mean that large quantities of meat are good for us. When I eat meat—which I only do about once a week, as is the Mediterranean way—I still like to be adventurous, and I like to offer adventurous choices to the diners in my restaurant, too. I offer free-range duck with orzo and figs, pecan and rosemary–crusted venison, or rabbit braised with Jack Daniels and prunes. I often serve lamb, which is common in Mediterranean cuisine, because it is a tender, flavorful, low-fat meat and because I can get fresh lamb right here in Maine. I also offer fish from local waters as an alternative to the ubiquitous salmon and grouper. I serve guinea hen or poussin instead of the standard chicken, and I even have a recipe for fried quail eggs. Not everybody jumps at these choices—people like to eat what they know—but courageous eaters can always find something exciting in my restaurant.

When I eat meat, I practice portion control. Nobody in the Mediterranean would think of eating a 16-ounce steak. Ridiculous! *Io non capisco.* Not only is meat expensive, but it is very filling and stays with you for a long time. You don't need very much to feel satisfied. I eat maybe 4 ounces, as a balance to the grains and vegetables that make up the rest of the meal. I still think of meat as something special, a pleasure and an indulgence, not something to binge on, let alone feature as the main source of food.

Decades ago in the Mediterranean, women and their families couldn't afford to indulge in meat every day, and thank goodness. Nutritionists studying the diet of the Mediterranean back in the 1950s credit the emphasis on plant foods with the area's extremely low disease rates and high longevity. Just because we may be able to financially afford to live on hamburgers and filet mignon doesn't mean we can physically afford to eat that way. I wouldn't want to eat that way, either. These foods certainly aren't my only love.

It all comes down to moderation. I'm all for pleasure. Food should fulfill us, indulge us, please us, and bring us into sensual harmony with the natural world. But the only way this works is if we remain balanced in what we take in. Rich animal foods — even lean animal foods — are just a part of the great abundance and variety of foods available to us.

These recipes include meat, poultry, fish, or eggs as just one part of a beautifully composed dish with a variety of colors, textures, and plant foods.

Charred Lamb Salad

Serves 4

Tender, flavorful lamb charred crispy on the outside and medium-rare on the inside makes vinaigrette-dressed salad greens into a hearty meal. The spices make this salad taste like something out of the eastern Mediterranean and make the small amount of lamb ultimately satisfying. Serve this salad with toasted pita or crusty bread. The pomegranate seeds add a nice crunch and crisp acidity to this salad. Try them as a garnish on other salads and grain dishes, too.

1 teaspoon sweet paprika

1/2 teaspoon hot chili powder

Pinch of cayenne pepper

1/4 teaspoon ground cinnamon

1/4 teaspoon ground cumin

1/4 teaspoon ground coriander

1/2 teaspoon salt

1/4 teaspoon black pepper

4 boneless lamb chops or cuts from leg of lamb, about 5 ounces each

1 tablespoon extra-virgin olive oil

1 tablespoon chopped fresh mint

1 tablespoon chopped fresh cilantro

1/2 cup shaved carrots

1 red bell pepper, cored, seeded, and cut into thin strips

8 cups mixed greens

Vinaigrette of choice, such as Chile-Lime Vinaigrette (recipe follows)

Pomegranate seeds for garnish (optional)

1. Mix the paprika, chili powder, cayenne, cinnamon, cumin, coriander, salt, and black pepper together. Set aside.

2. Preheat the oven to 400°F. Also preheat the grill on medium-high, or heat a cast iron or heavy sauté pan on medium-high.

3. Rub the lamb with the olive oil, then roll each piece in the spice mixture to coat. Char on the grill, marking both sides, or in the pan, about 2 minutes on each side.

4. Transfer the lamb to a baking pan and bake in the oven for 10 minutes. Set aside to rest.

5. In a large bowl, toss the mint, cilantro, carrots, bell peppers, and greens with the vinaigrette. Slice the lamb and arrange on top of the salad. Garnish with pomegranate seeds, if using.

Chile-Lime Vinaigrette

Makes about 1 cup

This tangy, spicy vinaigrette enhances the rich mild lamb flavor and blends in an interesting way with the mint and cilantro in the salad itself. You can use it to dress any salad, particularly when you want to match rich flavors in other dishes. It tastes great on crisp vegetable slaws. Try it over shredded cabbage and carrots with celery root and scallions, or with shaved raw vegetables.

1/4 cup rice wine vinegar

1 teaspoon sugar

2 peperoncini chiles, cored, seeded, and minced

Freshly squeezed juice from 1 large or 2 small limes

Salt and pepper to taste

1/2 cup extra-virgin olive oil (optional)

1. Heat the rice vinegar, sugar, and chiles in a small saucepan over medium-high. When the mixture begins to boil, remove from the heat.

2. Stir in lime juice and season with salt and pepper. Use like this, or whisk in the optional olive oil.

Grilled Tenderloin of Beef

with Iowa Blue Cheese Potato Gratin, Caramelized Cipollini Onions, and Porcini Mushrooms

Serves 4

This meal sounds fancy and complicated, but it's really just steak and potatoes with mushrooms and onions—a familiar American meal. The Mediterranean twist comes in the agro-dulce flavoring of the onions (that classic Mediterranean combination of sweet and sour), fresh mushrooms, and the addition of blue cheese to the potato gratin. You don't have to use Iowa's Maytag blue cheese—you can use any blue cheese you can find near you. Fresh crumbly goat's milk or sheep's milk cheese would work, too. You can make the gratin ahead of time and re-heat it.

FOR THE FILETS

4 filet mignons, about
*   5 ounces each*
2 tablespoons extra-virgin olive oil
Salt and freshly ground pepper to
*   taste*

FOR THE MUSHROOMS

1 pound fresh porcini, portobello, or
*   shiitake mushrooms, threaded on*
*   skewers*
2 tablespoons olive oil
Salt and pepper to taste
Freshly squeezed juice of 1 lemon

FOR THE ONIONS

2 tablespoons olive oil
1 pound cipollini or pearl onions, peeled
2 tablespoons unsalted butter
Salt and pepper to taste

FOR THE GRATIN

4 large Yukon Gold potatoes
1 cup heavy cream, milk, or chicken
*   stock*
1/2 cup crumbled Maytag blue cheese
Salt and pepper to taste
1 teaspoon chopped fresh thyme or
*   chopped chives*

FOR THE FILETS

Preheat the grill to high or preheat the broiler. Rub the filets with the olive oil and season with salt and pepper. Grill to desired doneness, about 4 minutes on each side for medium-rare. (You will also be grilling or broiling the mushrooms at the same time.)

FOR THE MUSHROOMS

Brush the mushrooms with the olive oil. Season with the salt and pepper. Grill the mushrooms along with the filet until grill-marked and tender, about 10 minutes. Finish with a sprinkling of lemon juice.

FOR THE GRATIN

1. Preheat the oven to 400°F. Peel and slice the potatoes so that the slices are about ⅛ inch thick.

2. Place the potato slices in a bowl with the heavy cream, blue cheese, salt, pepper, and thyme. Toss gently to coat well.

3. Layer the potatoes in a baking dish or deep cast iron skillet. Cover with foil. Bake for 45 minutes, then check the tenderness of the potatoes; bake longer if necessary.

4. Remove the foil and bake 15 more minutes, or until the top is golden brown.

FOR THE ONIONS

1. Preheat the oven to 400°F. Heat the olive oil in a heavy ovenproof skillet. Add the onions and cook until caramelized, 4–5 minutes. Add the butter and season with the salt and pepper.

2. Place the skillet in the oven and bake until soft, 10–20 minutes, turning the onions occasionally.

TO ASSEMBLE

Divide the gratin between four plates. Top each gratin with a filet, then garnish with the onions and mushrooms. Serve with a large green salad or wilted greens.

Guinea Hen Risotto

in Honey-Roasted Acorn Squash

Serves 4

Risotto is comfort food. This unusual version is flavored with guinea hen and is served in sweetened acorn squash decorated with vegetables. This meal is easier to prepare than it sounds, although it takes a little time. If you can't find or don't want to use guinea hen, you can substitute chicken legs, or even rabbit legs. You can also substitute finely grated good-quality Parmesan cheese for the pecorino.

FOR THE ACORN SQUASH

3 tablespoons honey

3 tablespoons unsalted butter

2 acorn squash, halved and seeded

Salt and pepper to taste

1/4 teaspoon nutmeg

FOR THE GUINEA HEN

4 guinea hen legs or chicken legs

Salt and pepper to taste

1 onion, peeled and chopped

2 stalks celery, trimmed and chopped

1 carrot, peeled and chopped

2 tablespoons tomato puree

3 garlic cloves, smashed

2 cups dry white wine

2 sprigs fresh thyme

2 bay leaves

1 teaspoon peppercorns

1 quart chicken stock or broth

FOR THE ACORN SQUASH

1. Preheat the oven to 400°F. In a small saucepan over low heat, combine the honey and butter until melted.

2. Put the squash in a roasting pan. Brush the squash with about half the honey butter. Season with the salt, pepper, and nutmeg.

3. Bake the squash for 25 minutes, or until tender. Remove from the oven and brush immediately with the remaining honey butter.

1. Heat a sauté pan over medium heat. Season the guinea hen legs with salt and pepper. Sear them on both sides until they are golden brown. Remove from the pan and set aside.

2. Preheat the oven to 350°F. In the same pan you used for the guinea hen, add the onions, celery, and carrots, stirring constantly until they begin to caramelize.

3. Add the tomato puree and garlic. Continue cooking and stirring, 4–5 minutes.

4. Add the wine and mix well, scraping up any bits from the bottom of the pan. Add the thyme, bay leaves, peppercorns, and stock. Bring the liquid to a boil, then reduce the heat so that the liquid simmers. Allow it to simmer for 5 minutes.

5. Place the guinea hen legs in a baking pan. Cover with the simmering liquid, then cover the pan with foil. Bake until tender, approximately 1–1½ hours.

6. Remove the guinea hen legs from the liquid and set aside. Strain the sauce back into the saucepan and continue to cook over medium-high heat until it is reduced by one-third, about 10 minutes.

7. Pull the meat from the leg bones and set aside.

FOR THE RISOTTO

1 quart chicken stock or broth

2 tablespoons extra-virgin olive oil

¼ cup unsalted butter

1 onion, peeled and chopped

1 garlic clove, peeled and minced

14 ounces Arborio rice

1 cup dry white wine

2 bay leaves

Guinea hen meat pulled from bones from previous directions

1 carrot, peeled, blanched in boiling salted water for 3 minutes, and diced

1 pound fresh spinach, roughly chopped

1 tablespoon chopped fresh thyme

3 tablespoons grated pecorino cheese

Salt and pepper to taste

1. Put the stock in a large saucepan and heat on medium until it simmers. Keep it at a simmer.

2. In a separate large saucepan over medium heat, combine the olive oil and 2 tablespoons of the butter. Add the onions and cook until soft but not brown, about 5 minutes. Add the garlic and cook 2 more minutes.

3. Add the rice and stir until it is coated with the fat. Pour in the wine and cook until the liquid is evaporated, about 15 minutes.

4. Add the hot stock 1 cup at a time, cooking while stirring constantly until each addition is completely absorbed. Once half the stock has been added, stir in the bay leaves, guinea hen meat, carrots, and spinach, and continue cooking and adding stock until the liquid is absorbed. This whole process should take 30–40 minutes.

5. When all the stock has been absorbed, remove from the heat and stir in the thyme, pecorino, and the remaining 2 tablespoons butter. Season with salt and pepper.

TO ASSEMBLE

Put each squash half on a plate. Fill each one with an equal portion of risotto and drizzle the sauce (prepared along with the guinea hen) over the top. Serve hot.

Merguez

This spicy sausage originated in North Africa but is also popular in France. Shaped into small patties, merguez makes a good appetizer or can be part of a meze platter. For a meal, serve this with couscous, pita wedges, and a crisp green salad or stuff them into pita bread halves topped with cucumbers, scallions, lettuce, and plain yogurt or Mint Yogurt (page 43).

½ pound lean ground beef

½ pound ground lamb

1 teaspoon salt

¼ teaspoon freshly ground black pepper

Pinch of cayenne pepper

Pinch of crushed red pepper flakes

1 garlic clove, peeled and finely minced

1 teaspoon ground cumin

1 tablespoon tomato paste

1 tablespoon harissa (optional, a spicy Tunisian condiment)

½ cup water, or as much as needed

1. Combine all the ingredients in a stand mixer with a paddle or with your hands. Add more or less water to get a consistency you can easily form into patties.

2. Form the meat into small patties, about 2 inches in diameter.

3. Heat a cast iron skillet or heavy sauté pan over medium heat. Cook the patties in batches until done, about 5 minutes on each side. Serve warm.

Pomegranate-Glazed Pork Tenderloin

with Honey, Ginger, and Cardamom–Scented Sweet Potatoes

Serves 2

This recipe adds fruit and sweet-potato spiciness to pork in the Mediterranean-African tradition. It's perfect for an intimate dinner with very little effort. These instructions tell you how to cook the pork in the oven, but you can also cook it on the grill with excellent results. You can use pomegranate molasses right out of the jar in place of the Pomegranate Glaze.

FOR THE POMEGRANATE GLAZE

3 pomegranates, or 1 cup pomegranate juice

½ cup sugar

1 tablespoon red wine vinegar

FOR THE PORK

1 tablespoon extra-virgin olive oil

1 pork tenderloin, 10–12 ounces

Salt and pepper to taste

⅔ cup chicken or beef stock or broth

1 tablespoon unsalted butter

½ cup pomegranate seeds (optional)

FOR THE HONEY, GINGER, AND CARDAMOM–SCENTED SWEET POTATOES

2 medium sweet potatoes

2 tablespoons unsalted butter or extra-virgin olive oil

1 tablespoon minced fresh ginger

½ teaspoon ground cardamom

1 tablespoon wildflower honey

Salt and pepper to taste

FOR THE POMEGRANATE GLAZE

1. Seed the pomegranates and push them through a mesh strainer, reserving the juice. Discard the pith. (If you are just using the juice, ignore this step.)

2. Place the pomegranate juice in a small saucepan with the sugar and vinegar. Turn the heat to high and bring to a boil,

then reduce the heat. Simmer for 10 minutes, then remove from the heat and set aside to cool. You will use about half of the glaze on the meat and about half for the final assembly.

1. Preheat the oven to 400°F. Heat a large cast iron skillet or a heavy ovenproof sauté pan over medium-high heat. Add the olive oil.

2. Season the pork with salt and pepper. Sear the pork in the pan on all sides, then place in the oven. Cook to 120°F internal temperature—this takes about 10 minutes, but use a meat thermometer to be sure. It could take longer.

3. When the meat is cooked, brush all sides with half of the pomegranate glaze. Return to the oven for 6 more minutes, and stop to glaze a few more times. Let the pork rest 4–5 minutes on a platter.

4. Meanwhile, add the chicken or beef stock to the pan and scrape up any browned bits. Whisk in the butter and season with salt and pepper. Set this sauce aside.

FOR THE HONEY, GINGER, AND CARDAMOM-SCENTED SWEET POTATOES

1. Preheat the oven to 400°F. Pierce the sweet potatoes and bake for about 1 hour, or until tender.

2. Cut the baked sweet potatoes in half. Scoop the pulp into a bowl.

3. Heat a sauté pan over medium heat. Add the butter or olive oil. When it is hot (about 3 minutes), add the ginger and cook 2 minutes. Add the cardamom and cook 1 minute. Remove from the heat.

4. Add the ginger mixture to the sweet potatoes. Stir in the honey and season with salt and pepper, smashing while mixing. If the potatoes are ready before the pork, keep warm until the pork is ready.

TO ASSEMBLE:

Mound the sweet potatoes on the center of a plate. Slice the pork tenderloin into about 10 slices. Arrange the sliced pork around the potatoes and drizzle a little pomegranate glaze around the plate. Pour the pan sauce over the meat and garnish with the pomegranate seeds, if using.

Braised Rabbit alla Cacciatore

This classic Italian dish is perfect for Sunday dinner when you have time to spend preparing something really special. The meat is braised in a rich concoction of high-flavor summer vegetables and olives. If you don't want to try rabbit or it's not available, you can easily substitute chicken legs. Use the leg quarters with the thigh attached. I like to serve this dish tossed with gnocchi, with the whole mixture on a bed of wilted greens. Try Wilted Swiss Chard (page 194), or sauté spinach quickly in olive oil with minced garlic until just wilted.

1 teaspoon mustard seeds

1 teaspoon black peppercorns

2 sprigs fresh tarragon

1 tablespoon chopped garlic

1 cup dry white wine

4 rabbit legs or chicken leg quarters

2½ tablespoons extra-virgin olive oil

Salt and pepper to taste

Flour for dredging (about 1 cup)

1 medium onion, peeled and chopped

1 stalk celery, trimmed and chopped

1 medium carrot, peeled and chopped

½ cup green olives in brine (preferably large Sicilian), drained, pitted, and chopped

½ cup gaeta or kalamata olives, pitted and chopped

2 garlic cloves, peeled and chopped

1 tablespoon tomato puree

1 cup crushed tomatoes

2 cups rabbit or chicken stock or broth

4 sprigs fresh rosemary (2 picked from stem, chopped and reserved; 2 whole for braise)

2 bay leaves

1 tablespoon unsalted butter

1 cup diced fresh mushrooms: portobello, crimini, porcini, or domestic,

2 plum tomatoes, seeded and chopped

1 tablespoon chopped fresh thyme

1. In a large bowl, combine the mustard seeds, peppercorns, tarragon, garlic, and white wine. Add the rabbit or chicken legs and turn to coat in the marinade. Let them marinate at room temperature for 3 hours or in the refrigerator overnight.

2. Heat a large skillet over medium-high heat and add the olive oil. Take the rabbit or chicken legs out of the marinade and season with salt and pepper. Reserve the marinade. Dredge the meat in flour (shake off excess). Place the rabbit or chicken in the skillet and brown on all sides. Do not overcrowd the pan.

3. Preheat the oven to 325°F. Put the meat in a casserole dish. Keep the skillet ready.

4. Add the onions, celery, carrots, and olives to the skillet. Cook until the vegetables are browned, about 10 minutes. Add half the garlic and cook another 2 minutes. Add the tomato puree and crushed tomatoes and brown carefully without scorching, about 5 minutes.

5. In a separate small saucepan, heat the marinade you used for the meat over medium-high heat until it is reduced by half, about 15 minutes. Add the marinade to the tomato mixture along with the stock, scraping up any browned bits.

6. Pour the tomato mixture over the rabbit or chicken in the casserole dish and top with the whole rosemary sprigs and bay leaves. Cover and bake for 2 hours. The meat should be falling off the bone. If it isn't, keep baking and check every 15 minutes.

7. Put the meat on a platter and pull it off the bones. Set the meat aside. Remove the rosemary sprigs and bay leaves, and puree the sauce with an immersion blender, or in small batches (carefully!) in a blender or food processor. Strain the sauce through a fine-mesh strainer, pushing on it with a spoon to get as much sauce as possible. Set aside.

8. Heat the skillet again over medium heat. Add the butter. When the butter begins to foam, add the mushrooms and cook until they soften, about 5 minutes. Add the rest of the garlic and the plum tomatoes and cook 2 more minutes. Add the vegetable sauce, the chopped rosemary, and the thyme. Add the rabbit or chicken meat and bring the whole mixture to a boil. Boil for 2 minutes, then ladle over hot pasta or gnocchi and toss to coat. If you wish, you can serve on a base of wilted greens.

Munchkin Pumpkins with Shrimp and Couscous

Serves 4

This dinner is easy to make but very impressive, so it's a fun meal to serve to friends or on special occasions. Kids will love using the mini pumpkins as bowls.

FOR THE COUSCOUS

1 cup couscous

1 tablespoon curry powder

1 cup hot water

1 carrot, peeled and chopped

3 tablespoons dried currants

Salt and pepper to taste

FOR THE PUMPKINS

4 mini pumpkins (about
    5 inches in diameter)

1 quart water or fish stock

4 carrots, peeled and chopped

1 large piece of ginger, peeled and
    chopped

1 garlic clove

1 bay leaf

1/4 cup chopped fresh cilantro, plus
    more for garnish

1 medium onion, peeled and chopped

1 serrano or jalapeño pepper, split in
    half

2 tablespoons unsalted butter

12 Gulf shrimp, peeled and deveined

Pumpkin seeds toasted in 300°F oven
    for 30 minutes, for garnish

FOR THE COUSCOUS

1. Place the couscous in a bowl. Stir in the curry powder, then add the hot water. Set aside and let the couscous "bloom" (swell until it has absorbed all the water). This should take about 15 minutes.

2. When the couscous has bloomed, add the carrots and currants and mix well. Season with salt and pepper.

1. Cut the tops off of the pumpkins to expose the seeds. Scoop out the seeds.

2. Place the pumpkins and tops in a large pot with the remaining ingredients, except for the shrimp and garnishes, over high heat. Heat to a boil.

3. Turn the heat down to medium-low and simmer the pumpkins until they are tender but not falling apart, about 15 minutes. Remove from the heat and strain the broth. Set the broth aside.

4. Preheat the oven to 400°F. Stuff three shrimp into each pumpkin. Place the pumpkins in a shallow casserole and add ½ cup of the broth to the casserole. Bake until the shrimp are done, about 10 minutes.

5. To serve, mound the couscous into four shallow bowls. Place a pumpkin on top. Replace the tops on the pumpkins. Pour the broth around. Garnish with chopped cilantro and toasted pumpkin seeds.

Quick-Cooked Salmon

with Fall Vegetable Pistou

Serves 4

Pistou is the French version of Italy's pesto—both include fresh basil, garlic, pine nuts, cheese, and olive oil to make a savory green paste. This recipe gives salmon a Mediterranean flair. You can use different vegetables or make your pesto with arugula instead of basil—whatever is fresh.

3 garlic cloves, peeled

1/2 cup pine nuts

1/2 cup finely grated pecorino or Parmesan cheese

1 cup plus 1 tablespoon extra-virgin olive oil

1 cup fresh basil leaves

2 cups vegetable or fish stock or broth

2 carrots, peeled and diced

2 parsnips, peeled and diced

1 cup broccoli florets (immerse in boiling water for about 2 minutes to blanch)

1 cup cauliflower (immerse in boiling water for about 2 minutes to blanch)

1 cup cooked fava, soy, or cranberry beans (or use canned, drained and rinsed)

2 cups new or fingerling potatoes, boiled until tender, drained, and diced

1 tablespoon extra-virgin olive oil

20-ounce wild Alaskan salmon fillet

Salt and pepper to taste

1. Make the pesto: Put the garlic in a food processor and process until well minced. Add the pine nuts, cheese, and 1/2 cup of the olive oil, and pulse until well ground. Add the basil leaves and 1/2 cup more olive oil, and puree until smooth. Set aside.

2. In a large saucepan, heat the stock over high heat. Add the carrots, parsnips, broccoli, cauliflower, beans, and potatoes. Bring to a boil, then turn down to simmer.

3. Swirl the pesto into the vegetable mixture a little at a time, reserving a little for garnishing at the end. Remove from the heat and set aside.

4. Put the remaining 1 tablespoon of olive oil in a sauté pan and heat on high until the oil ripples and just begins to smoke. Season the salmon with salt and pepper and place the fish, presentation side down (the side you will want up when you serve it), into the pan. Give the pan a quick shake immediately, then do not move until the salmon looks crispy on the edges, about 5 minutes.

5. Carefully turn the salmon and sear on the opposite side. Cook until the desired doneness. (I like to serve this rare to medium-rare, which takes about 5 more minutes.) Put the salmon on a platter and cut into 4 equal pieces.

6. Pour the pistou-vegetable sauce into four shallow bowls and place a piece of salmon on top of each. Garnish with a dollop of the pistou.

Spaghetti with Calamari all'Arrabiatta

Serves 4 to 6

Calamari, or squid, isn't a seafood commonly consumed in the United States except in its deep-fat fried form in restaurants. It is much more popular in the Mediterranean, where you can get it fresh from the sea. It really is delicious, so if you have access to fresh calamari where you live, try this delectable dish. If you can't find good calamari, you can substitute fresh clams or shrimp for a different but equally good taste. You can also top this with crunchy toasted bread crumbs instead of the cheese.

1 tablespoon salt plus more to taste
1 pound spaghetti
2 tablespoons extra-virgin olive oil
1 medium onion, peeled and diced
1 red bell pepper, cored, seeded, and diced
1 jalapeño pepper, cored, seeded, and diced
2 garlic cloves, peeled and minced
1 teaspoon crushed red pepper flakes
3 tomatoes, blanched in boiling water for 5 minutes and peeled

1 cup diced pickled cherry peppers (sweet or hot, find these with the pickled vegetables in the store, or substitute marinated red pepper strips)
1/2 cup chopped fresh Italian parsley
1 tablespoon chopped fresh oregano
Pepper to taste
1 1/2 pounds cleaned calamari

1. Bring 4 quarts of water to a boil over high heat in a large pot or Dutch oven. Add the 1 tablespoon salt, then the spaghetti. Cook 8 minutes, or until al dente. Drain and set aside.

2. Meanwhile, heat the olive oil on medium-high in a medium sauce pot. Add the onions, red bell peppers, and jalapeño peppers.

Madonna of Moderation
~ 173 ~

Cook until the onions are translucent, about 5 minutes. Add the garlic and red pepper flakes. Cook 2 more minutes.

3. Add the whole peeled tomatoes and pickled peppers and cook another 15–20 minutes. Add the parsley and oregano and check the seasoning, adding salt and pepper if necessary or some of the vinegar from the cherry peppers if you want a piquant sauce.

4. Using a tomato or potato masher, crush the tomatoes and peppers together. If you don't have a masher, use a food processor or a blender, but pulse only. You don't want a smooth puree.

5. Add the calamari to the sauce and heat it through, about 3 minutes.

6. Add the pasta to the sauce. Toss to coat. Serve hot, garnished with grated Parmigiano Reggiano cheese, accompanied by a crusty baguette and red wine.

Even if you are still hesitant about straying from your normal course of chicken breast and salmon fillet (those American protein staples), I hope you will try something new for your once-a-week meat indulgence. Be daring. Go gastronomically wild! Why not? Participate in the adventurous spirit of Mediterranean eating. If you live near the coast, find out what seafood comes fresh from the waters nearest you. If you live in the heartland, consider bison instead of beef now and then, or guinea hen instead of chicken. Try lamb for a change, or pork, or even rabbit or duck! Remember, variety keeps your meals interesting, expands your taste intelligence, feeds your body better, and tempts you to eat less by making every bite alluring. Just keep your servings small, eat meat only once a week, and you can try anything. Come on, I dare you. Live a little. *Comme les méditerranéens.*

9

To the Table, Famiglia

Eating at the family table was such an important part of my childhood and one of the ways in which my family most closely resembled the typical close-knit Italian families living in small towns along the Mediterranean coast. Dinner was a priority. We all sat down together and enjoyed several courses of good, fresh, home-prepared food. We began with an antipasto platter. We had soup, pasta, a fish course, a meat course, salad and cheese, and even dessert. We didn't argue about it, we didn't schedule things to do during this time, and we didn't fail to show up at the table. We just accepted dining as one of the requirements of living in a family.

✳ Making Time for Family

Of course, American women today sometimes have a hard time getting their partners and children together at the family table, let alone finding the time to prepare a meal worthy of such a gathering. The longstanding tradition in Mediterranean families seems like a luxury to many of us. But you don't have to be like the majority. Do you really want to be overweight, low on energy, and too busy to pay attention to the people you love and the food you eat? To really embrace the Mediterranean way of eating, you must embrace the Mediterranean way of living, which means making time for family and friends a nonnegotiable priority. Mediterranean women are more than just sexy and vital femmes fatales; they are also *madonnas*, life partners, and devoted mothers! Love of family and home is an earthy sensuality that is simply a part of who women are in the Mediterranean and how they live.

This may sound idyllic to you. But, hey, life isn't perfect. Maybe your family squabbles at the table, or the kids complain about the food, or nobody will come to the table even after you've proclaimed, "Dinner's ready!" three or four times. I know! Especially before everyone has embraced the habit of regular family dinners, establishing this time together can be difficult. But the effort is well worth the final result. You and your family will remember these dinners for the rest of your lives. I know I remember mine.

The argument I hear the most for not having regular family dinners is that people just don't have enough time, or they aren't all home from school or work or other activities at the same time. Women, men, and even our children take work very seriously in this country, even if that work is school or sports or volunteering. But Mediterraneans take family time, social gatherings, and mealtime very seriously. Their respect for family and food is a lesson for all of us.

Food is the most primitive form of comfort.
—Sheilah Graham, journalist

✳ Enjoying Food Without Gaining Weight

You might wonder what sitting down at the table with your family has to do with staying slim or losing weight. Step back a few feet and you'll see the big picture. It's all connected: taste, quality, freshness, and sharing that wonderful food with people you love. If you eat food under happy, warm circumstances with those you love, you will be so fulfilled in other ways that you won't need to stuff yourself for reasons that have nothing to do with physical hunger. Making a commitment to spend time at the table with family helps to bring all these elements together.

A close-knit family sharing food together, supporting each other, and expressing their fondness and love for each other makes life easier, less stressful, and more, well . . . filling. Good food may bring you all together and be the resource you share, but the big picture—all the pieces of a fulfilling, happy, pleasurable life—is bigger than what is on your plate today or tomorrow. The bigger picture is what brings you—your mind and your body—into harmony with yourself and the world around you.

What you are *not* doing when you eat with your family is very important. You aren't eating alone! Think about how you eat when you eat alone, or on the run, or in the car. Do you notice the food, or do you gulp it down as fast as you can and move on to the next thing? Do you eat way too much? Do you eat to numb your feelings when nobody is watching how much you are eating? The foods we eat in this informal and often alienated fashion tend to be less healthy, less fresh, and more processed, and we tend to eat much more than we need. But there is more to eating right than quality.

When you sit down at a table, use dishes and silverware, and eat food that you or someone you love has prepared, eating becomes an entirely different experience than when you eat in the car on the way from one place to another. When you focus on your food and the people you are sharing it with, you notice what you are eating. It tastes better. Each bite means more and fulfills you more. It may even nourish you more, as you are eating in relaxed surroundings with a positive mindset.

When you eat at the table and make mealtime an event, you may end up eating less, even if you are eating multiple courses. Just keep your portions small—just a taste! You will certainly feel more like you've really eaten and are less likely to want to eat again before the next meal.

In the Mediterranean, mealtime means conversation, each component of the menu a cause for celebration, discussion, and even analysis. Enjoying your food with others makes it a more vivid experience. What do you like? Why? What do your friends and family like? What are the differences in your preferences? Does one of you particularly appreciate the silky soup while another prefers the garlicky aroma of the pasta sauce? And do you note that hint of tarragon, or is it basil?

> *To lift off the cover of a tomato-y mixture and let it bubble up mushroom and basil under my nose does a lot to counteract the many subtle efforts a part of me makes to punish myself for all those worst of my shortcomings.*
>
> **—Mary Virginia Micka, poet**

People in the Mediterranean rarely eat alone because social participation is considered a crucial part of the dining experience. Food is for sharing. If you have a meal planned with your friends or family, don't waste your precious stomach space snacking first. Don't eat while you are cooking except to taste for seasonings. Let the meal be an event for you, whether it is a holiday or not. If you can manage at least one sit-down family dinner each week, consider it a triumph of the modern world. Cook for those you love, or let them cook for you. Sit. Savor. Eat! And make every bite worthwhile. Here are some ideas to help you share food with your friends and family.

Sean Kelly's Rosemary Roasted Almonds

Makes 4 cups

These almonds are easy to make and have so much more flavor than the salty canned almonds you can buy in the store. This recipe comes from my friend and Denver-based fellow chef Sean Kelly. Try a handful of this healthful snack food when you are hungry between meals to fill you up instead of making you even hungrier like high-carb snacks do. You can store these almonds in an airtight container for up to two months. These are also excellent served with sherry or any before-dinner aperitif, or with cheese, or as part of an antipasti, which you'll read more about later in this book.

4 cups unsalted raw almonds, with skins

1/2 cup extra-virgin olive oil

3 tablespoons chopped fresh rosemary

Salt and pepper to taste

1 teaspoon finely minced garlic

1/2 teaspoon crushed red pepper flakes

1. Preheat the oven to 350°F. Place the almonds on a baking sheet and bake for 20 minutes until they are lightly toasted but not brown. Meanwhile, place the rest of the ingredients in a large bowl and stir to combine.

2. Add the hot nuts to the bowl and toss to coat thoroughly. Taste and add more seasonings if necessary. Serve warm or at room temperature.

Classic Fondue

Fondue is a fun family activity as well as a filling meal if you include plenty of variety in the elements you use for dipping — whole-grain breads, raw or steamed vegetables, and juicy fruits. Use the very best cheese and good wine. Fondue makes a good holiday dish. You might make it a family tradition. If you don't have the kind of fondue pot that you can move on and off the burner, make the fondue in a saucepan first, then transfer it to the preheated fondue pot. Or you can put the fondue in a heatproof ceramic bowl in a stand over a candle flame.

1 garlic clove, peeled and halved

1 pound freshly grated Gruyère cheese

½ pound freshly grated Emmental cheese (or a good Swiss cheese)

1½ cups dry white wine (such as Neufchâtel)

1 teaspoon freshly squeezed lemon juice

4 teaspoons cornstarch

1½ tablespoons kirsch or other brandy

Freshly ground black pepper to taste

Pinch of nutmeg (fresh grated is best)

Dipping items of choice, such as cubed bread, bread sticks, toasted baguette slices, boiled purple and red bliss potatoes, red pepper strips, cucumber spears, apple slices, pear slices, pineapple spears, celery sticks

1. Use an unglazed fondue pot. Rub the inside of the pot with the garlic.

2. Combine the cheeses, wine, lemon juice, and cornstarch in the pot.

3. On the stove over medium heat, stir with a wooden spoon in a figure 8 motion until the cheese melts. Stir in the kirsch, pepper,

and nutmeg. Cook, stirring occasionally, until smooth and creamy, then transfer the pot to a fondue burner.

4. Serve with a variety of dipping items. Be sure to stir as you dunk!

Artichokes with Lemon Aioli

Artichokes are so unusual in appearance and in the way they are eaten that they can seduce even itinerant vegetable haters. The tender flesh is really irresistible. Placing several artichokes at different spots on the family table for people to share is a sure conversation starter as everyone compares their opinions on this spiky vegetable and takes turns tearing off the leaves and dipping them. When you get to the hairy-looking choke, scrape it off and pare it away to reveal the heart, which can then be divvied up for happy consumption. You can serve a variety of dips with artichokes—as simple as olive oil and lemon juice, melted butter with lime juice, or tomato sauce, or as complex as a fancy French béarnaise sauce. I like this tangy lemon aioli, a favorite Mediterranean condiment that is so much nicer than mayonnaise.

4 medium artichokes	1 teaspoon coriander seeds
1 cup dry white wine	1/2 teaspoon black peppercorns
Freshly squeezed juice of 1 lemon	5 garlic cloves, peeled and smashed
2 bay leaves	1 cup extra-virgin olive oil
1/2 cup chopped fresh basil leaves	Lemon Aioli (recipe follows)

1. Preheat the oven to 400°F. Prepare the artichokes: Cut off the top thorny tip (about 1 inch from the top) using a serrated knife, and cut off the bottom of the stem. Pull off the tough outer leaves. Trim the outer layer of skin around the bottom with a sharp paring knife.

2. Place the artichokes upside down in a deep casserole dish and add the rest of the ingredients except the lemon aioli, plus

enough water to cover the artichokes. Cover and bake until the bottoms are tender and easily pierced with a fork, about 1 hour.

3. Remove the artichokes from the baking pan and serve each artichoke with a dollop of lemon aioli or use it on the side as a dipping sauce.

Lemon Aioli

Use this classic French condiment instead of mayonnaise. You'll never go back. It is also delicious on cold fish, cold meat, hard-boiled eggs, and grilled vegetables. If you can find Meyer's lemons, they make an excellent aioli, but any fresh lemons will do.

3 egg yolks

1 tablespoon Dijon mustard

Zest of 2 lemons

3 garlic cloves, peeled and finely minced

1½ cups extra-virgin olive oil

2 tablespoons freshly squeezed lemon juice, plus more if needed

Salt and white pepper to taste

1. Process the egg yolks and Dijon mustard together in a food processor. Stir in the lemon zest and garlic.

2. Slowly drizzle in some of the olive oil as the food processor is running. When the mixture thickens slightly, begin alternating a few drops of the olive oil with a few drops of the lemon juice, until the aioli is the consistency of mayonnaise.

3. Season with salt and pepper. If the aioli is too thick, add more lemon juice. If it tastes too acidic, thin it with a little water. Store in a covered jar in the refrigerator for up to 1 week.

Yellow Velvet Soup

In the Mediterranean, a soup course is often served between the appetizer course and the pasta course. You can use this soup as a course or as the centerpiece of the meal with a big salad. Fresh-picked ingredients make this soup extra special. The heavy cream adds to the velvety texture, but plain milk will make a less filling soup that will still taste good. I don't use olive oil in this soup because it could overwhelm the delicate flavors—canola oil is a good, mild alternative with similar health benefits to olive oil.

1½ tablespoons canola oil	1½ teaspoons minced garlic
1 medium onion, peeled and diced	1 bay leaf
2 small or 1 large yellow squash, peeled and diced	1 quart vegetable stock or broth
	½ cup heavy cream or milk
4 sweet corn ears, kernels cut off the cob	Salt and pepper to taste

1. Heat the canola oil in a large saucepan or soup pot over medium heat. Add the onions and cook until translucent, about 8 minutes. Add the squash and corn, cooking 4–5 more minutes, stirring occasionally. Add the garlic and bay leaf, cooking 2 more minutes.

2. Add the vegetable stock and bring the soup to a boil. Turn the heat down to medium-low and let the soup simmer until all the vegetables soften, about 10 minutes.

3. Add the cream and bring the soup back to a boil. Season with salt and pepper. Remove from the heat and cool slightly, remove the bay leaf, and then puree with an immersion blender, or in small batches in a regular blender or food processor.

4. Strain the soup through a large-holed sieve. Taste and add more salt and pepper if necessary. Serve warm.

Pasta Alla Puttanesca

This is pasta sauce "harlot" style, a robust southern Italian tomato sauce usually made with tomatoes, garlic, chile peppers, capers, olives, anchovies, and oregano. The reference to prostitutes supposedly suggests this was a sauce quickly made between clients. It is most often associated with Naples and Calabria, although versions are found throughout Italy (and for that matter, the United States). Harlots notwithstanding, this is a great sauce for Americans who may be similarly rushed in their daily schedules, even if for different reasons! Enjoy it as a pasta course for a big family dinner or as the main course.

1 tablespoon extra-virgin olive oil

5 garlic cloves, peeled and chopped

1 teaspoon crushed red pepper flakes

4 plum tomatoes, chopped

2 cups tubular pasta

Salt to taste

3 cups tomato sauce

1 cup gaeta, niçoise, or kalamata olives, pitted and chopped

4 tablespoons capers

10 fresh or canned anchovy fillets, rinsed, patted dry, and chopped

1 tablespoon chopped fresh oregano

Pepper to taste

Caperberries for garnish, optional

1. Heat the olive oil in a large skillet over medium heat. Add the garlic and cook 2 minutes, but do not brown. Add the red pepper flakes and tomatoes, and cook 2 more minutes.

2. Meanwhile, cook the pasta in boiling salted water according to package directions.

3. Add the tomato sauce, olives, 2 tablespoons of the capers, and the anchovies to the skillet. Cook for a few minutes until the flavors begin to meld together. Add the oregano, salt, and pepper. Serve over the hot pasta and garnish with the remaining 2 tablespoons capers or caperberries.

To the Table, Famiglia

Atlantic Salmon and Green Garlic

Baked in Parchment Paper with Fine Herbs

Serves 4

The idea of a fish course after pasta and soup and before a meat course, cheese course, and dessert sounds a little overwhelming to most Americans, but remember that in the traditional Mediterranean each course is very small and the family cook might spend most of the day preparing the meal. Most of us don't have the time for that sort of thing. This dish makes a perfect feature and takes just enough time to prepare that you feel you really put forth an effort to produce a quality meal. It's fun to unwrap the little paper packets to reveal the salmon redolent with green garlic. Serve with a big salad, crusty bread, and a light red table wine or a rich white wine for a complete menu — although the soup or pasta course in this chapter would be nice to serve first, if you are so inspired.

4 sheets parchment paper (at least 12 × 12 inches)

4 wild or organically farm-raised salmon fillets, about 6 ounces each

4 stalks green garlic, thinly sliced (if you can't find green garlic, substitute 4 small leeks or scallions, tops and bottoms)

4 tablespoons dry white wine

4 teaspoons extra-virgin olive oil

Salt and pepper to taste

1 cup chopped fresh chervil, parsley, chives, and tarragon

4 teaspoons unsalted butter

1. Preheat the oven to 400°F. Fold each sheet of parchment paper in half, and cut a heart shape approximately 3–4 inches bigger (when folded in half) than your salmon fillet.

2. Unfold the parchment and place a fillet near the fold. Place a handful of green garlic next to it. Drizzle each fillet with wine

and olive oil, then sprinkle with salt, pepper, and herbs. Top with a pat of butter. Fold the edges of the parchment paper up tightly.

3. Place the paper packets on a baking sheet and bake 10–15 minutes, or until the parchment paper is puffed and slightly brown. Remove from the oven and open carefully onto dinner plates, allowing the steam to safely escape. Serve hot.

Lentil Roast

Serves 4

Many Mediterranean meals are vegetarian, not because the people living in the Mediterranean have an aversion to meat, but because meat is considered a luxury. This hearty loaf, reminiscent of meat loaf, is made mostly of plant foods. It is delicious, warming, and comforting. Best of all, you will feel light and energetic after eating it rather than weighed down. Serve with Parsnip Mashed Potatoes (recipe follows), your favorite grilled or sautéed vegetables, and a salad.

1 cup red lentils

2 cups vegetable stock or broth

1 bay leaf

2 teaspoons dried whole-wheat bread crumbs

2 cups grated sharp cheese, such as sharp Cheddar

1 leek, finely chopped

4½ ounces mushrooms, finely chopped

1½ cups fresh whole-wheat bread crumbs

2 teaspoons chopped fresh parsley,

1 teaspoon freshly squeezed lemon juice

2 eggs, lightly beaten

Salt and pepper to taste

1. Preheat the oven to 375°F. In a large saucepan, combine the lentils, vegetable stock, and bay leaf. Bring to a boil, cover, and reduce to a gentle simmer for 15–20 minutes, or until the liquid is absorbed. Remove from the heat. Remove the bay leaf and set aside.

2. Sprinkle the dried bread crumbs into a 9 × 5 × 3-inch loaf pan.

3. Stir the cheese, leeks, mushrooms, fresh bread crumbs, and parsley into the lentils. Combine the lemon juice and eggs in a small bowl and beat well. Stir them into the lentil mixture and combine thoroughly. Season with salt and pepper.

4. Spoon the lentil mixture into the loaf pan and smooth the top. Bake for 1 hour. Slice and serve.

Parsnip Mashed Potatoes

These are sweeter and more interesting in flavor than plain mashed potatoes. Use milk instead of cream if you want a lighter version. You can also use olive oil instead of butter for a slightly different flavor.

1½ cups Yukon gold or yellow fin
    potatoes, peeled and cut into
    chunks
1 pound parsnips, peeled and cut into
    chunks

1½ cups heavy cream or milk
3 tablespoons unsalted butter
Salt and pepper to taste

1. In two separate saucepans, boil the potatoes and the parsnips until each is fork-tender. Drain and put both together in a mixing bowl with a whip attachment. Set aside.

2. In a medium saucepan, combine the cream and the butter over low heat. When the butter is melted, turn on the mixer and whip the potatoes and parsnips on low speed. Add the cream–buttter mixture a little at a time to the potato–parsnip mixture until all is added and you have a thick, creamy consistency. Season with salt and pepper and serve hot.

Mustard Crusted Lamb Chops

with Roasted Fingerling Potatoes and Wilted Swiss Chard

Serves 4

Lamb is popular in the Mediterranean but is not served nearly as often as beef in the United States. This recipe pairs rich, tender lamb chops with a tangy, crunchy mustard crust. Add fingerling potatoes and wilted Swiss chard for a complete and delicious dinner without too much effort. Everyone will feel well tended, even the cook.

4 lamb chops, 6–8 ounces each
    (4 ounces for boneless chops)
Salt and pepper to taste
2 eggs
2 teaspoons whole-grain mustard
1 teaspoon Dijon mustard

1 cup dried bread crumbs
3 garlic cloves, peeled and minced
2 tablespoons chopped fresh Italian
    parsley
2 tablespoons extra-virgin olive oil

1. Preheat the oven to 400°F. Season the lamb chops with salt and pepper. Set aside at room temperature.

2. In a bowl, mix the eggs with the mustards, and season with salt and pepper.

3. In a separate bowl, mix the bread crumbs with the garlic, parsley, and 1 tablespoon of the olive oil. Season with salt and pepper.

4. Put the remaining 1 tablespoon olive oil in a heavy skillet over medium-high heat. Sear the lamb chops until they are brown on all sides. Remove from the pan and let sit 3–4 minutes to cool.

5. Brush each chop with the egg mixture, then dredge in the bread crumb mixture. Place the chops on a rack over a baking sheet or roasting pan and bake until browned, 7–10 minutes. Serve with roasted fingerling potatoes and wilted swiss chard (recipes follow).

Roasted Fingerling Potatoes

Fingerling potatoes are very popular in restaurants lately, but you can substitute any small potatoes that look good.

1½ pounds fingerling, red, or yellow fin potatoes, halved	1 tablespoon chopped fresh rosemary
3 tablespoons extra-virgin olive oil	2 garlic cloves, peeled and minced
	Salt and pepper to taste

1. Preheat the oven to 400°F. Toss the potatoes with all the other ingredients.

2. Put the potatoes on a baking sheet. Roast for 30 minutes, or until tender.

Wilted Swiss Chard

This versatile and high-nutrition wilted chard makes the perfect bitter contrast to rich meats such as lamb and beef. You can substitute other greens, too—collards, beet greens, kale, spinach, or whatever looks good.

1 bunch fresh Swiss chard (red, white, or rainbow)

2 tablespoons extra-virgin olive oil

3 garlic cloves, peeled and minced

1 teaspoon crushed red pepper flakes

Salt and pepper to taste

1 tablespoon unsalted butter

1. Tear the Swiss chard leaves from the ribs and wash them well (they tend to be sandy). Pat them dry with paper towels.

2. Heat the olive oil in a large skillet over medium-high heat. Add the garlic and cook 2 minutes, but do not let it brown.

3. Add the red pepper flakes and chard. Season with salt and pepper, then add the butter. Let the chard wilt, turning it while it cooks, 4–5 minutes. Drain on paper towels and serve.

Fruit Sorbet

Serves 4

A multicourse meal doesn't need a fancy or rich dessert. Fruit sorbet is just right, as a refreshing sweetness after a light meal. I don't suggest ever feeling guilty about anything delicious you decide to eat, but you certainly won't feel guilty about this dessert. The sweetness and flavor come almost exclusively from the fruit. You can use any fresh fruit puree. Just cut ripe fruit into pieces (remove pits) and puree in the food processor with a little water or juice until smooth. (Peeling the fruit first is optional, except for mangoes.) This recipe gives you some suggestions and shows you approximately how much fruit it takes to make 4 cups of puree.

4 cups fruit puree (see directions above)
1¼–2 cups simple syrup (equal parts water and sugar, simmered over low heat until the sugar is dissolved — use 2 cups for a sweeter sorbet or when using a tarter fruit)
1–2 tablespoons freshly squeezed lemon juice
1–2 tablespoons liqueur such as kirsch, Grand Marnier, or Frangelico
Pinch of salt

1. Mix all the ingredients to taste. Whisk well and chill overnight, or for at least 3 hours.
2. Churn according to your ice-cream machine directions.

Fruit Equivalents

Mangoes: Approximately 7 mangoes equal 4 cups puree.
Peaches: Approximately 4 pounds equal 4 cups puree.
Apricots: Approximately 3 pounds equal 4 cups puree.
Plums: Approximately 3 pounds equal 4 cups puree.

Whether your family dinners are simple or complicated, quick and easy or several courses long, I urge you to implement this tradition in your home. Even if you live with just one other person, sit down together as often as you can. If you live alone, invite friends or family over to share meals with you at least a few times every week. If you meet friends or family in a restaurant, you are still sharing food together, eating with laughter and love, and building memories. It will be worth every bite, worth every moment.

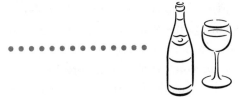

10

Water and Wine

In the Mediterranean, eating is very important, but so is drinking—drinking water and drinking wine. Although some Mediterranean countries do not drink wine, to many—including France, Italy, and Spain—wine is more than just a beverage; it is an integral part of meals and an essential aspect of social gatherings. Water, too, is essential to life—anywhere of course, but Mediterranean women drink water all day long. Let's look at these two vital beverages and a few others while considering how they might help you get more vitality out of your life and even how they can help you stay slim.

✳ Water, Water Everywhere...

Water is life. We are made up largely of water and cannot live long without it. Water is in almost everything we eat and drink, but in its pure unadulterated form, it is one of the most powerful weight-loss tools you have at your disposal. Drinking plenty of water every day makes your kidneys work more efficiently to flush waste from your body. It gives you more energy, it keeps your skin glowing, and it helps your whole body work better.

Most American women don't drink enough water. We take a bottle to the gym with us or drink it in restaurants, but many people don't drink it throughout the day. What a waste! Instead, many of us get our "water" from beverages such as coffee and diet soda. When you make water your main beverage and drink it all day long, you don't get any of the calories, chemicals, or caffeine in other beverages. Water is so easy to drink and so wonderful for your body. Do you know why you don't drink it? Because you aren't in the habit! The more water you drink, the more you will enjoy it and even crave it. And the more you will learn to tune in to your body's cues that it needs water.

Drinking water is the most natural thing in the world. If you can make it your quintessential beverage—always defaulting to water except on special occasions or for a rare treat—your body will feel so much better, and chances are you'll lose weight more quickly. Women in Europe drink water throughout the day, but they don't carry a bottle with them wherever they go. They don't drink water on the run, in the car, or while walking down the street. Throughout the day (and by now, this probably won't surprise you), women living in the Mediterranean stop what they are doing, pour themselves a refreshing glass of water, sit down, and drink it. Yes, when Mediterraneans drink water, they really drink water. They pay attention to what they are doing. When they are finished, they move on with their day. What a great way to enforce little breaks into your day, to stop your body and your brain from their normal crazy pace and just relax into the full attention of drinking the earth's most precious and life-bestowing beverage.

Women in Europe tend to drink their water at room temperature rather than ice cold. Some believe ice-cold water is bad for digestion. I like my water closer to room temperature, too, as it goes down more smoothly. Cold dulls the taste of most foods, and a really great mineral water is better at a higher temperature because you can appreciate its subtleties.

But it doesn't matter what kind of water you drink, as long as it is clean and pure. If you don't like water, try mineral water, which adds trace nutrients and tends to have a silkier mouth feel and more flavor. A wedge of lemon will help cleanse your body with natural citrus. (Those "flavored" waters are more likely to contain artificial sweeteners and other additives with no nutritional benefit.) You might even try a "water tasting" with different brands of spring water and mineral water. When you really tune in, you might be surprised at how different waters taste from each other.

Experts recommend different amounts of water, although the standard you have probably heard is that most women should drink eight to ten glasses of water each day. That's about one-half gallon each day. Most women don't have trouble drinking that much water if they just make it a habit. You don't need to drink any more than that. Fill up a gallon jug with purified water every other day and finish it in two days (keep it on the counter if you like it at a higher temperature, or in the refrigerator). You'll be tapping into one of the secrets of how Mediterranean women stay so slim, strong, and healthy.

☀ Aperitivo

People in Italy wouldn't think of ingesting a big meal without first preparing their system for food with an *aperitivo*. This before-dinner drink might be a "martini," which in Italy is simply a glass of vermouth—hold the gin or vodka. Or it might be a nice moscato d'asti—a sweet, sparkling wine—or a glass of

Madeira. Dubonnet with soda, French vermouth, Byrrh, Cointreau, the light, fruity Lillet, or a small glass of cognac might precede a meal in France. Champagne is another wonderful before-dinner drink, especially for celebratory meals.

Spanish sherry is more likely to warm the stomach before dinner in Spain. Typically, these little drinks are served in very small amounts and are sweet, so they don't appeal to everyone. But women in the Mediterranean don't doubt the important digestive influence of these beverages. They don't add a lot of calories or an intoxicating influence because portions are so small. Just a few ounces to put you not only in the right physical state for digestion but in the right state of mind, easing you out of your workday into the friendly, sociable state best for sharing a meal with the people you love.

To practice this tradition, you certainly don't need to drink liquor if you don't want to. Nevertheless, I urge you to practice the tradition of preparing for the meal physically and mentally. Many people use their juicers to prepare before-dinner cocktails of fresh juice, no alcohol required. Try a concoction such as carrot-orange, apple-celery, or banana-pear. The most important thing about an *aperitivo* is that it be small and lightly sweet or gently dry, or even a little bitter, to get those digestive juices flowing. Sit. Enjoy your cocktail, whatever it is. Clear your mind and refocus on the meal to come rather than the work of the day.

❋ Wine and Food: A Heavenly Pairing

In some Mediterranean countries, wine is not a part of regular life, but in the western Mediterranean, particularly in Spain, France, Italy, and Greece, a meal without wine is like . . . well, it isn't much like a meal! The pairing of wine and food is truly ancient in this part of the world. The Greek harvest goddess

Demeter is also the goddess of wine and agriculture, which has long been the livelihood of the Mediterranean region.

The way women drink wine and other drinks in the Mediterranean is very much in the spirit of the harvest and the table—much different than the way most people drink them here in the United States. Wine is filled with ritual and tradition. It is thought to mingle with foods in a very particular way and, most importantly, it always goes with food. People in the Mediterranean would never stand around at a party drinking wine all night without eating food! That's not how it works at all. *Claro que no!*

In the Mediterranean, women typically have one small glass of wine with dinner, and that means about 4 ounces! Not much compared to the big bowl-shaped glasses brimming with wine we tend to drink in the United States. Hundreds of studies have demonstrated the positive effect of moderate wine consumption on heart health, stress levels, blood pressure, and even longevity. The key is moderation. Just a little bit and *always* with food. That's the Mediterranean way. It's also the way to enjoy the great health benefits of wine without subjecting yourself to too many calories from alcohol or (and this is important) alcohol's tendency, when consumed in excess, to make the drinker eat much more than she really needs.

What is it about moderate wine consumption that is so healthful? Some people believe it is the plant compounds found in red wine, while other studies demonstrate equally beneficial effects from white wine and even from liquor and beer consumption—but always, of course, in moderation.

Muslims in the eastern Mediterranean most certainly do not drink alcohol, yet still enjoy good food and good health. If you don't drink or don't want to drink with every meal, that is, of course, perfectly fine. I don't drink wine every day. Daily drinking isn't nearly as much a part of our culture as it is in the western Mediterranean, where even children sometimes get spoonfuls of wine in their water glasses.

> *In France, wine is thought of as food, so necessary to life that nobody is too poor to go without it.*
>
> — **Katharine Butler Hathaway, writer**

✳ What to Drink

Matching wine with the right food can make or break a great recipe. First courses of antipasto or soup might be served with a crisp white wine such as Sauvignon Blanc or Pinot Grigio. Pasta with red sauce goes well with a light red table wine, while pasta in a light cream sauce or tossed with fresh vegetables and olive oil blends perfectly with a rich Chardonnay.

Forget the traditional idea that white wine must go with fish. If seafood makes up your main course, try a flowery Pinot Noir or a fruity Cabernet Franc or Sangiovese. Choose white wines such as Chenin Blanc or Pinot Gris for light, delicate fish in subtle sauces. Meaty red wines such as Cabernet Sauvignon, Zinfandel, and Syrah have the strong character to make a perfect foil for rich meat dishes such as lamb, beef, and rabbit, while lighter reds and whites work well with poultry and lean cuts of red meat lightly dressed in delicate sauces. If you don't drink, consider matching fresh-squeezed or purchased organic purple and white grape juices with your meal or other juices from interesting fresh fruits. Or consider matching your meals with different herbal iced teas or even varieties of mineral water, a tasting experience on its own.

The only way to really figure out which wines you like and what tastes good with your favorite recipes is, of course, to taste, taste, taste. Keep a journal and list the wines you've tried, what foods you tried them with, and how they tasted to you at the time. The more you taste wine, the more you will learn to appreciate its subtle nuances and the way it can bring out the flavors in one dish while obliterating the flavors in another.

> *Wine is earth's answer to the sun.*
> — **Margaret Fuller, writer**

Wine tasting is an adventure, but it is not meant to be a drunken one. In the Mediterranean, a glass of wine is only about 3 or 4 ounces, not the 8- to 12-ounce portions you tend to get in the United States. Each little taste of wine goes with each little taste of food in a beautiful marriage of flavor. Binge drinking isn't healthy, and drinking wine in the Mediterranean has nothing to do with overconsumption. *Mettere la testa a posto!* (Make sure your head is on straight!)

Between courses, you needn't dirty every wineglass in the house, either. Choose a good, basic wineglass shape with room to swirl the wine around, releasing the aroma for a full sensual appreciation before you take a sip, then fill up your glass with water between each glass of wine to cleanse your palate, rinse out your glass, and stay well hydrated throughout the meal.

Wine is often used in cooking in the Mediterranean, too. Try a splash of wine in a pasta sauce, as a replacement for vinegar in a salad dressing (this is a good way to use wine that is past drinking when you didn't finish the bottle), to flavor or marinate meat or fish, to give an added depth and complexity to soups, and even to flavor desserts such as custards and cookies. I'll share some of my favorite recipes that use wine and spirits later in this chapter.

> *Cheese that is required by law to append the word food to its title does not go well with red wine or fruit.*
>
> **— Fran Lebowitz, writer**

✳ *Digestivo*

Finally, no meal is complete without a *digestivo*. While the *aperitivo* is sweet, the *digestivo* tends to be bitter—so bitter that some people have a hard time even tasting them. They are definitely an acquired taste. But in the Mediterranean, the *digestivo* is just as important as any other course of the meal. The bitter taste helps to settle the stomach and promote healthy digestion. This is incredibly important to the Italians, and they will be glad to talk to you for quite a while about the state of their own digestion!

After the final salad and cheese courses, a tiny glass of bitter grappa may be the quintessential Italian *digestivo*. This distilled wine is made from the bitter stems and other residue from the grapes after winemaking, and it has a harsh taste. A bitter lemon limoncello is a somewhat milder but still effective *digestivo* that is also popular in Italy. We make our own at Primo (see page 207). Other *digestivos* include Fernet-Branca, a walnut liqueur called Nocino, good port, robust sherry, Vin Santo or marsala, and Sambuca. Licorice, citrus rind, nuts, and other deep bitter flavors work best to wind down the celebration of sharing food and drink with friends and family.

You can find the same bitter digestive-aiding qualities in herbal teas. We make our own herbal teas at Primo, and we have an extensive tea garden full of herbs. Your local markets probably stock many different types of teas. Ginger, licorice, chamomile, cinnamon—all these are warming and slightly bitter or pungent digestive aids that will help you to relax and unwind after a meal, sharing a warm cup with friends and reflecting on your gastronomic experience.

Incorporating these drinking traditions into your life will help you to appreciate, even cherish, every meal and every coming together of family and friends in a way that is not only Mediterranean but ancient and venerable. Celebrate your food. Celebrate the harvest. Raise your glasses in a toast: *Cin Cin!*

☀ Homemade Stuff

Making homemade liqueurs is easy and fun to do. Make them about six weeks ahead of when you want to serve them, or keep them in your pantry all the time. You can use sterilized Mason jars for aging, then pour the finished liqueur into attractive bottles you have saved from purchased wine and spirits. Just be sure the bottles are washed in very hot, soapy water and dried with clean towels, or run them through the hot cycle on your dishwasher.

Sweet Orange Aperitivo

Makes about 4 cups

This sweet, enticing before-dinner drink will help to whet your appetite before dinner. Use organic oranges without blemishes, and cut off any moldy, bruised, or soft spots. Nonorganic oranges are often dyed and waxed, and they could have trapped pesticides in the skin.

4 organic oranges
1 vanilla bean
1 cinnamon stick
2 cups vodka

1 cup brandy or cognac
1 cup sugar
1 cup water

1. Wash the oranges well, then cut them into wedges. Remove the seeds.

2. Put the oranges, vanilla bean, and cinnamon stick in a sterilized glass jar. Add the vodka and brandy. Cover and steep in a cool, dark place for 2 weeks.

3. After 2 weeks, take the jar out. Combine the sugar and water and boil over high heat until the sugar is completely dissolved, about 5 minutes. Add this sugar syrup to the jar. Return the jar to a dark place and age for 4 more weeks.

4. When the liqueur is done aging, strain it through a wire mesh strainer into a clean glass bottle. Serve in small glasses at room temperature or over ice.

Primo Limoncello

Try this lemon liqueur as a *digestivo*. It is a very popular after-dinner drink in Italy and easy to make at home. Keep it in the freezer—it tastes best when it's very cold. If you don't cut the pith from the peel, this will be very bitter, so try to get most of it off with a sharp knife. Use organic lemons so that you aren't adding dye, wax, and chemicals to your lovely liqueur.

1¼ cups lemon peel (cut off all signs of the white pith)
2 cups vodka

1 cup sugar
1 cup water

1. In a large saucepan, add 1 cup of the lemon peel and pour the vodka over it. Store the remaining lemon peel in the freezer.

2. Heat the vodka and lemon peel over low heat until the vodka is just barely warm. Remove from the heat and pour the mixture into a sterilized glass jar. Cover and store in a cool, dark place for 1 week.

3. After 1 week, combine the sugar, water, and remaining ¼ cup frozen lemon peel in a small saucepan over high heat. Bring to a boil and cook until the sugar is completely dissolved, about 5 minutes.

4. Strain the lemon peel out of the vodka mixture and put it in a large glass measuring cup. Strain the lemon peel out of the lemon syrup and add the syrup to the vodka mixture. Mix well and pour into a clean glass bottle. Store in the freezer and serve ice cold.

Amaretto

Makes about 3 cups

This liqueur is a lovely almond flavor with just a hint of bitterness. It makes an excellent *digestivo*, or it can be an *aperitivo*, depending on your mood. Try it drizzled over ice cream, or put some in your coffee. Or let it stand in for dessert, all on its own. If you use blanched almonds, the amaretto will be less bitter, but some people prefer some nutty bitterness.

1 cup sugar

1 cup water

1 cup raw unsalted almonds, roughly chopped

¼ teaspoon pure almond extract

3 cups vodka

1. Combine the sugar and water in a small saucepan over high heat. Bring to a boil and cook until the sugar is completely dissolved, about 5 minutes. Store half of this sugar syrup in the refrigerator until needed.

2. Put the almonds in a sterilized glass jar. Add the almond extract, vodka, and half the sugar syrup. Cover tightly and shake until thoroughly combined. Put the jar in a cool, dark place and allow to steep for 2 weeks.

3. Strain the amaretto through a fine mesh strainer to remove all of the almonds. Add the remaining sugar syrup and stir.

4. Age the amaretto for 3 more weeks, then serve at room temperature.

Tisane

Serves 4

Tisane is just a fancy word for herbal tea. We make herbal teas at Primo according to what herbs inspire us from our garden. You can experiment with your own combinations, too. This lemon-mint tisane is an excellent *digestivo* to help you process a delicious dinner. It can also stand in for dessert. To make other tisanes, just follow the same directions using your own combinations of fresh or dried herbs from your garden, farmers' market, or natural health food store. Always use organic herbs, of course. You want to make your tisane with the essence of the herbs themselves and nothing else. If you don't like your tea sweet, just leave out the honey, although it does coax the flavors from the herbs in a subtle way.

3 sprigs lemon verbena

1 sprig lemon balm

1 sprig mint

1 lemon, cut into thin slices

2 tablespoons honey

1 quart boiling water

4 sticks rock candy (optional, look for it in fancy candy stores or online)

1. Put the herbs and lemon in a clean glass jar or pitcher. I like to use 1-quart Ball jars.

2. Pour the boiling water over everything and let steep for at least 15 minutes. Strain through a fine-mesh sieve or coffee filter and serve warm or chilled over ice with honey to taste and a rock-candy stick.

Tummy Tamer Tisane

Serves 4

This tisane is perfect for when your digestion feels a little off. It can help settle your stomach or make you feel better if you are feeling nauseated. Use fresh or dried herbs, whichever you can find.

1 sprig calendula
1 sprig bergamot

1 sprig mint
1 quart boiling water

1. Put the herbs in a clean glass jar or pitcher, or a 1-quart Ball jar.

2. Pour the boiling water over everything and let steep for at least 15 minutes.

3. Strain through a fine-mesh sieve or coffee filter and serve warm.

✳ Food with Spirit

The rest of the recipes in this chapter are some of my favorite dishes that use wine and spirits. Consider these recipes as a guide for adding wine and spirits to your own dishes. I always use good wine rather than so-called cooking wines because the quality makes a difference.

Sherry Vinaigrette

Makes about 2½ cups

Wine and other spirits add an interesting depth to salad dressings. Try this sherry vinaigrette on your next green salad. Use a good Spanish sherry, not a cheap cooking sherry, and you will really notice how it enhances the flavor.

1 cup sherry vinegar	1 teaspoon honey
2 tablespoons balsamic vinegar	½ cup light olive oil or olive–canola
¼ cup dry Spanish sherry	oil blend
¾ cup minced shallots	Salt and pepper to taste

1. Combine the vinegars, sherry, shallots, and honey in a medium bowl.

2. Whisk in the olive oil a little at a time. Season with salt and pepper. Serve immediately over crisp fresh greens.

Braised Rabbit with Cracked Olives

Serves 4

Braises are dishes in which meat or poultry is cooked for a long time in liquid. They are the perfect opportunity for using wine because the wine gives the braise an added complexity, but the whole dish cooks for so long that all the alcohol cooks out. If you can't find or don't want to use rabbit, you can substitute a whole chicken instead. Both versions are delicious. Serve over linguine with Wilted Swiss Chard (page 194).

2 tablespoons extra-virgin olive oil

1 whole rabbit or 1 whole chicken, cut into pieces

Salt and pepper to taste

Flour for dredging

1 tablespoon unsalted butter

1 medium onion, peeled and roughly chopped

2 stalks celery, trimmed and diced

2 medium carrots, peeled and diced

6 garlic cloves, peeled and slivered

4 tablespoons tomato puree

1 cup dry white wine

2 cups rabbit or chicken stock or broth

1 cup Mediterranean green olives in brine (preferably picholine), smashed and pitted

4 sprigs fresh rosemary, leaves picked from the stems and chopped

One 28-ounce can whole peeled tomatoes, crushed, with their juice (I like Muir Glen)

2 bay leaves

1. Preheat the oven to 325°F. Heat a large ovenproof skillet with a cover over medium-high heat. Add 1½ tablespoons olive oil to the skillet.

2. Season the rabbit or chicken pieces with salt and pepper and lightly dredge them in flour. Sear the seasoned meat in the skillet until golden on all sides. Remove from the skillet and set aside.

3. Melt the butter in the skillet. Add the onions, celery, and carrots. Cook, stirring, until the vegetables are lightly browned, about 5 minutes. Add the garlic and cook 2–3 more minutes. Add the tomato puree and stir. Cook 3 more minutes.

4. Add the white wine and bring the whole mixture to a boil. Lower the heat to medium and cook, stirring occasionally, until the liquid is reduced in volume by about half, about 15 minutes. Add the stock, browned meat, olives and their brine, rosemary, tomatoes, and bay leaves.

5. Bring the entire mixture back up to a boil, then lower the heat to medium to simmer. Cover the pan and place in the oven for 2 hours, or until the meat is fork-tender.

6. Remove from the oven and take the meat out of the sauce. Put it on a plate and set aside. Skim any fat off the sauce. Remove the bay leaves. Serve the meat on a platter over linguine with the sauce ladled on top.

Tuna with Cabernet Whipped Potatoes

Wine and potatoes may seem like a strange combination, but this is one way to make your mashed potatoes taste really interesting. Serve with wilted greens tossed with a little red wine, or a fresh green salad dressed with the sherry vinaigrette from this chapter. These potatoes also complement fresh salmon steaks or fillets.

1 bottle (750 ml) Cabernet Sauvignon wine

1 teaspoon minced shallots

1 teaspoon minced garlic

Freshly ground black pepper to taste

1 quart heavy cream

1 pound Yukon Gold potatoes, peeled (or not) and boiled

Salt to taste

1 tablespoon extra-virgin olive oil

4 tuna steaks, about 5 ounces each

1. In a medium saucepan over medium-high heat, combine the wine, shallots, garlic, and freshly ground black pepper. Cook, stirring occasionally, until the volume is reduced to about one-fourth the amount you started with, 30–40 minutes. Stir in the cream and cook, stirring occasionally, until the sauce thickens slightly, about 10 more minutes.

2. Mash the potatoes by hand or put them through a foodmill. Stir in the wine–cream mixture and season with salt and pepper.

3. Heat a skillet over medium-high heat. Add the olive oil. Sear the tuna on both sides, leaving it medium-rare—about 3 minutes on each side. Remove from the pan and serve with the mashed potatoes.

Camembert with Zinfandel Poached Pears

Serves 4

In traditional Mediterranean celebratory meals, salad, cheese, and dessert courses often follow the meat course. This dish combines them all. Loganberries are a raspberry-blackberry hybrid — if you can't find them, just substitute raspberry or blackberry puree. Make berry puree by processing about 2 cups of berries with a little bit of juice or water in a blender or food processor.

1½ cups loganberry, raspberry, or
  blackberry puree (see directions
  above)
1 cinnamon stick
6 cloves
4 peppercorns
2 cups Zinfandel wine
2 cups water
½ cup sugar

4 firm pears, preferably Comice or
  Bosc, peeled and cored
½ pound mizuna (a lacy Japanese
  green, or substitute other fresh
  greens)
8 ounces Hudson Valley (or your
  favorite brand) Camembert, cut
  into 4 wedges

1. In a large saucepan, combine the berry puree, cinnamon stick, cloves, peppercorns, wine, water, and sugar. Bring to a boil over high heat. Add the pears and turn the heat down so that the liquid simmers.

2. Poach the pears at a simmer until they are tender, about 40 minutes. Remove the pears from the saucepan and cut each one in half from stem to bottom. Keep simmering the sauce to reduce it slightly, about 15 minutes.

3. Place a tuft of mizuna in the center of each of four plates. Place two pear halves on the greens, then top the pears with a wedge of cheese. Drizzle with the wine sauce and serve immediately.

Mediterranean Women Stay Slim, Too

Price's Port Cherry Sauce

Serves 4

Price makes a delicious cherry sauce with ruby port. Use fresh cherries if you can get them in season, but frozen will work, too. Try this over a small serving of gelato or ice cream, or stir it into yogurt or custard for a simple dessert.

1 cup ruby port   *1 cup pitted cherries*
1/2 cup sugar

1. Combine the port and sugar in a medium saucepan over medium-high heat, stirring until the sauce thickens, about 15 minutes.

2. Add the cherries and continue cooking 5 more minutes (10 minutes if the cherries were frozen).

3. Serve warm or at room temperature. Store in a glass jar in the refrigerator for up to 2 weeks.

Cooking with wine is just as fun and interesting as drinking wine with dinner, so I hope you will try it. From appetizer to dessert, wine and spirits make food livelier and add an intriguing depth of flavor. Plus, most or all of the alcohol cooks out when heated. I also hope you will learn how to drink wine in the Mediterranean spirit, if you like to drink it and your health allows for it. Remember the importance of portion control. Pour 4 ounces (1/2 cup) of wine into a glass and look at it. That's all you need in a day. Sip it slowly, savor it with your food, and sink into the pleasure of the experience. Combined with delicious food, that little bit can make every night's dinner a truly memorable experience.

11

Take It or Leave It

O mangier questa minestra o saltar questa finestra!
Either eat this soup or jump out this window!

I have to say that I find some of the American attitudes toward food a little strange. Women in particular seem to have a love-hate relationship with food, and we are teaching this love-hate food fight to our daughters. We fear our food, thinking it will make us fat or unhealthy. But yet we feel addicted to food and eat way too much of it. And the food we often choose to overeat is *bad* food—processed, fatty, tasteless. Food filled with chemicals or sitting in layers of plastic on a shelf for months. Food made with fake fat, fake sugar, fake color. No wonder this food fails to satisfy or nurture our inner goddess! *C'est mauvais pour la digestion!*

This way of eating is entirely foreign in Mediterranean culture, where people cherish quality, taste, and the sensual experience of eating. Emotional eating isn't Mediterranean, nor is bingeing. Sure, the food is so good that sometimes you want to eat a lot of it! But this happens within a broader, more balanced scheme. A day of luxuriously heavy eating is followed by a day of light, tasty food and walking a little more briskly. In Sicily or Rome, these brisk walks are called *passigata*.

The more-more-more concept seems to permeate American thinking, including attitudes about food. If one cookie is good, three are better. If one slice of pizza is good, three are better. Eat the whole 4-pound steak and you get it for free! Buy it in bulk! Supersize it! I know this is all familiar rhetoric to you, whether you subscribe to the ideas or not. But there is also a trend turning away from this attitude. Even some fast-food restaurants have decided to stop offering a "super" version of their meals. As more studies suggest that lower calorie consumption is linked to longer life, people are taking a second look—more is not always better. It's just more.

In its second season, according to an article published in the Australian *Herald Sun*, the luxury liner *Queen Mary 2* has already suffered the collapse of dozens of its seats, installed by a French company, due to the excessive weight of some passengers. The newspaper article specifically pins the seating collapses on "obese American passengers." While the French company, with typical French restraint, won't specifically say that Americans were the cause, we can only imagine that these seats were designed with a typical European customer in mind. Do we really want to be the cause of disintegrating furniture because we can't stop overeating? *Certainement pas!*

It isn't easy. Portion control is tough, and it can be even tougher to round up really good food conveniently. What do you do when faced with an all-American all-you-can-eat buffet for $10 or a tiny plate of high-quality food for $25? No, it isn't easy. Yet, it is possible. It's more habit than anything else, and breaking a habit is just breaking a habit; it's not changing your whole personality.

The Italians have a saying: *Mangia poco ma bene*. (Eat little, but eat well.) That is the single most important key to staying slim because you won't overeat, but you won't feel deprived, either. The Mediterranean diet offers you truly good food with relatively little effort, with such full flavor that small portions seem like plenty.

Over the years, I've come to some other conclusions about how to stay slim eating the Mediterranean way, and I'd like to share my top ten with you. Reorienting your thinking and your habits according to these ten Mediterranean-inspired ideas will help you to eat incredibly delicious food, really enjoy it, and stay or get slim because you are focusing on quality, not quantity. Will it be easy? Sometimes. But not always. Old habits are hard to break, even when the new ones fill you with pleasure. But you know what they say . . . *Pour faire une omelette, il faut casser des œufs!* (To make an omelet, you have to break a few eggs!) Here's how to direct your mind toward the Mediterranean:

1. *Become a food snob.* It's not that Mediterranean women are necessarily food snobs, but they know what quality is, and they don't waste time or calories on anything but good food. What's the point? I'm certainly not suggesting you turn your nose up at your friends, but that doesn't mean you can't turn your nose up at what they eat, especially if it is fast food, junk food, processed food, or poor-quality food with mediocre ingredients. Cultivating your inner food snob can actually be fun if you approach it in a lighthearted way. *No voglio quello, ringraziamenti per offrire!* (I don't want that, but thank you so much for the offer!)

2. *Be picky.* Kids are often picky about what they eat, refusing to eat things with flavors or textures they don't enjoy. The foods that American kids don't like are often the healthy choices—vegetables, fish, whole grains—but in the Mediterranean, where children grow up eating what the adults eat and refining their palates at a much younger age, pickiness is more about pleasure. Why eat something that doesn't fill you with pleasure? *Je ne sais pas.* Be picky and don't settle for food that doesn't infuse you with childish joy. Even if it's a healthy food such as fish or green beans or apples, don't eat it if it isn't well prepared and delicious. The food you eat should be truly good and worthy of your body (remember rule number 1!). If it isn't, just say, *No, grazie!*

3. Slow down. Americans always seem to be in a hurry. In general, life in the Mediterranean isn't about rushing through the day. It's more about savoring the day. You can carry this attitude into many aspects of your life. Take your time to look around and notice what you are doing, taste what you are eating, listen to who is talking to you, and pay attention to the world as it spins past you. Chew your food. Taste it. Don't just gulp and swallow. If you really tune in to the experience of every bite and enjoy each morsel of food in your mouth as long as possible before sending it into your stomach, you'll find that you don't eat as much. At the same time, your meals will be more memorable.

4. Shun fast food. This is the flip side of rule number 3. Slow down by shunning fast food. In the Mediterranean, food isn't fast. It might be convenient at times, it might be easy to make, it might be very simple, but fast? *Certainement pas!* One group in favor of this rule is Slow Food. This international organization works to combat the trend toward fast food and the homogenization of food by raising awareness about the positive benefits of knowing the origins of your food and preparing it with care, encouraging the practice of biodiversity, and funding initiatives devoted to taste education, gastronomic culture, and the preservation of traditional foods in danger of being lost to the world. Slow Food, founded by Carlo Petrini in 1986 (not surprisingly, he is an Italian), now has 80,000 members in 100 countries. If you want to learn more, chances are there is a local Slow Food chapter near you. Check the Internet at www.slowfoodusa.com.

5. Buy local. It is quintessentially Mediterranean to eat what grows where you live, and to know your growers, whether they are the people who run that little produce stand on the highway or the regulars at the farmers' market, or the butcher, baker, and produce clerk at your local grocery store. Let them know who you are, talk to them, ask them questions, and make it known that you are looking for the very best. It really does make a difference if you know where the food comes from. You will appreciate your food and treasure it much more. You'll be less likely to waste food or cook more than you need. You will also find yourself woven into a community if you cultivate these relationships. Plus, people are social creatures by nature, and they like it when others are interested in what they do. Show interest, and you might just get the inside scoop on when the best food will be available.

6. Go organic. In a world with a huge population and factory farms producing food in bulk, pesticides, herbicides, and chemical fertilizers seem to be a necessity for efficiency and profit. But many farmers are standing up and arguing with that so-called wisdom by practicing organic farming methods and sustainable agriculture. The result for consumers is food grown without chemicals or the lingering aura of environmental destruction. Dousing food in the substances used by American producers would be scandalous to many Mediterranean producers, and Mediterraneans wouldn't buy the stuff, anyway. When you choose organic food and free-range organic meat, you will not only be supporting these earth-friendly practices, but you will be getting food much closer to what you would get in the Mediterranean, where food is grown on small farms nearby and carted to the market immediately after picking. If you are getting to know your food producers, you might discover that many small farmers don't go through the huge expense to have their food certified organic, but that doesn't mean they don't use organic farming methods. Ask and they'll tell you. Our small farms and farmers, especially those practicing organics, are the caretakers of our land. They give back to the soil as they farm, keeping the land healthy and providing food with greater nutritional value.

7. *Pay attention to what you buy. Pay more for it.* Organic produce often costs more than "regular" produce in the grocery store (although it may actually be less at the farmers' market when it is in season and an even better value than produce in the supermarket). The more you taste the difference, the more you may realize that a few extra pennies are well worth the higher quality. You'll find that better-quality food generally costs more than processed food made with cheap ingredients. A jar of mass-produced pimiento-stuffed "Spanish" olives from California is a lot cheaper than a jar of artisanally produced olives like those from the Santa Barbara Olive Company, also based in California, but what a difference! Would you rather pay less for a wrapped-up slice of processed cheese food or more for a wedge of spectacular aged French cheese or a hunk of lovely fresh artisanally crafted sheep's cheese? You see what I mean. Sometimes paying more for quality food really is an investment in your health and in your own pleasure. You often get what you pay for, so pay attention to what goes into your basket and buy the food that you decide is worth eating.

8. *Exercise portion control.* Portion control may be one of the hardest things for Americans to get a handle on. It's just so easy to take more. We've got so much food available to us! But part of the beauty of cherishing and savoring your food is that less is more. What's so valuable about a pound of spaghetti with canned sauce? But half a cup of risotto studded with wild mushrooms and rich sauce, well . . . that's something entirely different. Have you ever noticed that the more expensive the restaurant, the smaller the portion size? And the cheaper, the bigger? In French, the phrase to have a hearty appetite — *avoir un bon coup de fourchette* — literally means to have a good way with the fork. It has nothing to do with huge portions; it has to do with a huge appetite for goodness, flavor, and quality. Keep your portions small and your food good, and you'll value every bite and feel more satiated.

9. *Follow the recipe.* One good way to help keep portions small is to follow the recipe. If a recipe says it serves four, don't eat the whole thing yourself. Divide it between four people, or eat one-fourth of it and put the rest in the freezer for later. Put the rest away *before* you start eating so that you won't eat mindlessly. Europeans are generally shocked by the portion sizes in American restaurants and homes — portion sizes that have grown substantially in the past few decades. Whether pasta, steak, wine, or one of those jumbo frozen drink glasses, our vision of what serves one person is getting pretty cloudy. So when you cook at home, follow the recipe and take the number of servings quite literally. Pay attention to a single serving. Then when you go to a restaurant, you will know how much of that jumbo plate of food to eat and how much to save for later.

10. *Follow the three-bite rule.* Another funny thing about American eating habits is the concept of "cheating." You ate a piece of cake or a cookie, and now you feel horribly guilty because you cheated. On whom? On what? Special treats should be special treats, but feeling guilty about them destroys all the pleasure and ruins the whole point of getting to enjoy a piece of cake or a cookie. Eating them every day isn't a good idea for anyone, but eating them every now and then when the opportunity for something truly good presents itself . . . well, that's just living life to the fullest! If you are following the other nine rules, you aren't going to be bingeing on packaged cookies or junk food, anyway, but when something excellent comes along—a fresh French pastry, a homemade birthday cake, a warm batch of chocolate chip cookies made by someone who loves you, a scoop of gelato—follow the three-bite rule. The first three bites of a new taste are always the best, so just take three luscious bites, and stop. Wasn't that a satisfying treat? *Ça descend tout seul!* No guilt allowed, or necessary.

I'll devote the remainder of this chapter to some of my favorite indulgences in which quality of ingredients is absolutely paramount. Make them with love and savor them with restraint, and you'll truly be living *la dolce vita.*

Candied Pecans or Walnuts

Makes 2 cups

A serving of these sugary nuts is about 1 ounce, or about an eighth of a cup. Use high-quality, fresh, raw nuts that are unsalted. Relish just a few in silence, and it will be a good day. Pass the rest around to your family. You'll probably get an empty bowl passed back to you. Nuts are high in fat but also high in protein and energy. A few go a long way, and they are great for your skin.

2 cups whole pecans or walnuts   *½ cup hot water*
1 cup light brown sugar

1. Preheat the oven to 375°F. Put the nuts on a baking sheet and toast them for 5–8 minutes, or until they turn a golden brown. Don't overbrown them.

2. Meanwhile, put the brown sugar in a medium bowl. Add the hot water very gradually, mixing well after each addition until the sugar looks like thick, wet sand. (You might not need all the water.)

3. Add the hot nuts to the sugar and stir well until all the nuts are coated. Turn them back out onto the baking sheet and bake an additional 5 minutes. Serve warm or at room temperature. Store in an airtight container for up to 2 weeks.

Summer Tomato-Feta Salad

with Tapenade Crostini

Serves 4

This beautiful salad makes a filling and luxurious lunch if you use a collection of freshly picked tomatoes from the garden or farmers' market, a good Greek feta or locally produced goat cheese, and Tapenade Crostini you make yourself. If you can find heirloom varieties of tomatoes, these make the salad even more special. I like Marvel Stripe and Big Daddy Sunburst.

2 yellow tomatoes, sliced
2 beefsteak tomatoes, sliced
1 pint pea shoots
1 pound feta cheese, broken into 4
   chunks

8–10 cherry tomatoes
Extra-virgin olive oil to taste
Sea salt and freshly ground black
   pepper to taste
Tapenade Crostini (recipe follows)

1. Assemble the sliced tomatoes on a plate. Arrange the pea shoots, cheese, and cherry tomatoes around the sliced tomatoes.

2. Drizzle the whole salad with olive oil. Sprinkle with sea salt and pepper. Garnish with the crostini.

Tapenade Crostini

Serves 4

8 baguette slices, cut about 1/4 inch thick

1 garlic clove, peeled and cut in half

1 cup pitted kalamata olives

2 teaspoons chopped garlic

1½ tablespoons capers

2 fresh or canned anchovy fillets, rinsed and patted dry

2 tablespoons chopped fresh basil

1 tablespoon extra-virgin olive oil, or more if necessary

Freshly squeezed juice of 1 lemon

Salt and pepper to taste

1. Preheat the oven to 400°F. Put the baguette slices on a baking sheet and toast in the oven until golden, about 10 minutes. Rub each toasted baguette with the garlic clove halves. Set aside.

2. Combine all the remaining ingredients in a food processor. Process until spreadable but still slightly grainy. Add more olive oil if the mixture is too stiff. Adjust the seasoning.

3. Spread the tapenade on the baguette slices and serve.

Fresh Sheep's Ricotta Frittata

with Mushrooms and Herbs

Serves 2

This recipe is plenty for two people for breakfast or lunch. Use fresh organic eggs produced locally, for maximum taste and nutrition, and a quality sheep's milk ricotta, or regular ricotta if that's all you can find. Don't bother with the low-fat ricotta, which has very little taste. Eggs and cheese may seem like an indulgence to the diet conscious, but this is a nutritious and heart-warming recipe that takes very little time to prepare. It also makes a great supper when you want to go without meat. Just cut this recipe in half to make yourself a nice meal when you happen to be on your own. You'll feel light and happy afterward.

1 tablespoon unsalted butter

1 cup sliced assorted mushrooms, such as domestic, portobello, shiitake, or chanterelle

1 tablespoon chopped fresh thyme

1 tablespoon chopped fresh rosemary

1 tablespoon chopped fresh sage

1 tablespoon chopped fresh parsley

Salt and pepper to taste

4 eggs

2 tablespoons sheep's milk ricotta (or regular ricotta)

1. Preheat the oven to 400°F. Melt the butter in an 8-inch non-stick ovenproof skillet (an omelet pan is perfect if you have one) over medium heat. Add the mushrooms and cook until tender, about 6 minutes. Add the thyme, rosemary, sage, and parsley. Season the mushrooms with salt and pepper.

2. In a small bowl, beat the eggs lightly. Pour them over the mushrooms, and scramble with a rubber spatula until almost

set. Smooth evenly over the bottom of the pan. Spoon small dollops of the cheese on top of the eggs.

3. Place the skillet in the oven for 3–4 minutes, or until the frittata turns puffy and lightly brown. Slide the frittata onto a cutting board and cut it in half. Serve with mixed fresh fruits for breakfast or a tossed salad for lunch or dinner.

Pasta with Tomato-Pepper Coulis

Serves 4

The low-carb craze says no to pasta, but just imagine what an Italian would say to such a notion. Life without pasta? *Pazzo*— that's crazy! Just keep your portion size to one-half cup. With this delicious sauce, you'll be glad you indulged in quality rather than quantity.

4 ounces pasta

2 tablespoons extra-virgin olive oil

1 medium onion, peeled and thinly sliced

1 tablespoon minced garlic

1 red bell pepper, cored, seeded, and sliced

6 plum tomatoes (overripe), halved

1/2 cup dry white wine

1 cup vegetable stock, chicken stock, or water

1 bay leaf

2 ounces shaved pecorino cheese

1. Cook the pasta according to the package directions.

2. Meanwhile, heat the olive oil in a large skillet over medium-high heat. Add the onions and cook, stirring, until translucent.

3. Add the garlic and cook 2 more minutes. Add the peppers and cook until softened. Add the tomatoes and cook another 2 minutes, stirring occasionally, then add the white wine and cook until all the liquid is evaporated, about 10 minutes.

4. Stir in the stock and bay leaf, and cook until the tomatoes are tender and the sauce thickens slightly, about 10 more minutes. Remove the bay leaf.

5. Using an immersion blender, puree the sauce, or puree in small batches in a regular blender or food processor. Pass the sauce through a sieve. Serve over the pasta. Garnish with the pecorino cheese shavings.

Fresh Corn Fritters

Serves 4 to 6

Fried food? Can you possibly eat fried food? Sure you can, if the ingredients are fresh, the food is fried quickly so that it doesn't absorb much oil, and you eat only a little. Indulgences like these aren't for every day, but one or two golden-brown corn fritters are okay once in a while. Serve these as a garnish to a big salad. They also pair beautifully with Yellow Velvet Soup (page 186).

1 cup fresh corn, cut from the cob
3 egg yolks, beaten
½ cup all-purpose flour

1 teaspoon chopped fresh marjoram
¼ teaspoon salt
About 1 cup canola oil

1. Put the corn in a large bowl and mash it with a potato masher or a fork.

2. Add the egg yolks, flour, marjoram, and salt, and thoroughly combine.

3. Fill a small skillet with deep sides with about 1 inch of the canola oil. Heat over medium-high. Carefully drop the batter in 1-tablespoon dollops into the hot oil. Cook for 2 minutes on each side. Drain the fritters on paper towels and serve immediately.

Ricotta Cheesecake

A small, perfect slice of ricotta cheesecake is one of life's great pleasures, and like other indulgences, certainly not for every day. But when life warrants a big celebration, try this recipe. Expect rave reviews. The ricotta gives the cheesecake a unique texture, lighter and airier than what you can get with cream cheese. You need to make the crust at least a few hours before you make the rest of the cheesecake, so plan ahead if you are making this recipe for a big event. The nice part about this crust is that you are making crumbs out of it, so you don't have to worry how it looks when you roll it out.

A note about the marsala in the filling: Marsala is an Italian fortified dessert wine. If you don't have any, consider purchasing a bottle. It makes a nice *digestivo* or stand-in for dessert, and it is very Italian. Dry marsala is lighter and makes a good *aperitivo*. Both are good to use in cooking, too, adding a sweet, smoky depth to food.

FOR THE CRUST

12 tablespoons unsalted butter

3/4 cup sugar

1 egg

1/4 teaspoon vanilla extract

1 1/2 cups all-purpose flour

3/4 teaspoon baking soda

1/4 teaspoon salt

FOR THE FILLING

1/2 cup golden raisins

1/4 cup sweet marsala

1/2 cup pine nuts

4 cups whole-milk ricotta

3/4 cup heavy cream or milk

4 large eggs

9 tablespoons sugar

Pinch of cinnamon

1/2 teaspoon vanilla extract

1/4 teaspoon almond extract

5 tablespoons all-purpose flour

1. In a large mixing bowl, combine 8 tablespoons butter and the sugar. Cream them together until light and fluffy.

2. Mix in the egg and vanilla extract, beating until smooth.

3. Sift together the flour, baking soda, and salt. Stir the dry mixture into the butter mixture until combined. Turn out the dough onto a sheet of plastic wrap and form it into a ball. Wrap it up and chill for 2 hours or overnight.

4. Preheat the oven to 350°F. Divide the chilled dough into two pieces. Roll each half out into a rectangle ⅛ inch thick.

5. Place the rectangles on a baking sheet and bake 10–15 minutes, until golden. Cool slightly and crumble them both. Place the crumbs in a bowl.

6. Melt the remaining 4 tablespoons butter and stir into the crumbs. Butter an 8½-inch round springform pan and press the crumb mixture onto the bottom and up the sides of the pan to form an even crust.

FOR THE FILLING

1. Preheat the oven to 350°F. Place the raisins in a bowl.

2. Heat the marsala in a sauté pan over medium heat. When it is hot but not boiling, pour it over the raisins. Let stand for 20 minutes to plump.

3. Meanwhile, spread the pine nuts onto a baking sheet and toast in the oven 2–3 minutes until golden but not dark. Set aside.

4. Place the ricotta, heavy cream, eggs, sugar, cinnamon, vanilla extract, and almond extract in a bowl. Sift the flour over the top and whisk the ingredients together for 4 minutes, or until well combined.

5. Add the plumped raisins with the marsala and the toasted pine nuts and mix well. Spoon the batter into the prepared crust.

6. Put the springform pan on a baking sheet and bake for 1¼ to 1½ hours, or until the top is golden brown and has puffed.

7. Cool on a rack for at least 20 minutes, then chill in the refrigerator for 1 hour. Run a spatula carefully around the sides and unmold. Enjoy one tiny, perfect slice!

Are you in touch with your inner food snob yet? I hope so! I really believe this is one of the easiest, most pleasurable, and quickest paths to weight loss. If it isn't quality, if it isn't absolutely irresistibly delicious, then why bother? It is important to snack often to keep your metabolism fueled, but shun that junk food and you'll be shunning pollution. You don't need to be "fancy" or "gourmet" to be devoted to quality. A juicy apple, a handful of unsalted cashews, a small cube of beautiful French cheese, a little dish of bright red pepper strips, a spoonful of savory hummus . . . quality snacking that fuels your body the right way. Because you deserve only the best. You're a goddess—like the Louvre's *Winged Victory*, take flight with confidence, strength, and style. You're fit to fly!

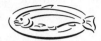

12

What's Good for Your Heart

Food may nourish the soul, but in many ways—both physically and emotionally—it also nourishes the heart. Your heart is your emotional center. Love may not literally flow from your heart, but humankind has decided to think of the heart that way for so many centuries that you may be tempted to think it's true. Even if it doesn't actually govern feeling, your heart does keep the lifeblood flowing through your body, making all the parts work, nourishing your muscles, feeding your brain, and flushing your cheeks when you really *feel* something. So perhaps the heart and the emotions are linked after all.

In the Mediterranean, heart disease rates have been among the lowest in the world. Unfortunately, this is starting to change as people eat a more Americanized diet. A diet of plant foods rich in olive oil with small amounts of red wine does wonders for the heart, but that isn't the whole story. Eating heart-healthy food can help you stay healthier longer and avoid chronic diseases, but it can also feed your heart in other ways. Sharing good food with the people you love is a way to express your love for them. Eating food produced locally helps you become connected in a meaningful way to your community. That sense of connection with others helps to lower your stress and make you feel better about your life, which is also very good for your heart.

I think that family closeness and coming together around the table does a lot to feed the heart and keep it healthy and strong. Mediterranean families stay together, and several generations may live together long past the time when American families have split apart and gone their separate ways. This emotional closeness and physical proximity throughout the years really does feed the heart by giving every family member a sense of place, belonging, and emotional support.

In the Mediterranean, another heart-healthy aspect of life is that famous tendency to vent emotions. Recent studies show that holding in anger and repressing feelings may actually damage the heart—and what loud, boisterous Italian family would disagree? Mediterranean women express their feelings and move on. They don't fret and stress about things without speaking up. They express themselves because they have a clear sense of who they are and what their role is. And they fall back into their loving relationships with the air perfectly cleared.

> *Educating the mind without educating the heart is no education at all.*
>
> **—Aristotle, Greek philosopher**

A friend of mine recently mentioned how much she loved Italy because she felt like a woman there. I asked what she meant, and she explained that men and women in the United States seem more confused about their roles. "Women often feel they have to act like men, so they forget how to act like women.

A lot of us earn the money, run our lives, and find ourselves in charge of other people, and suddenly we don't know what it means to be a woman anymore." My friend quickly explained that many women in Italy also earn money, run companies, and manage their own lives, but somehow they also seem to be very comfortable with themselves as women—and men respect them as women. "In Italy, men truly love and respect women for being women, and women have this beautiful sense of what it means to be a woman. They don't try to take on both roles. They can separate what they do from who they are."

Understanding who you are as a woman and embracing your feminine side doesn't mean being subservient or staying home while your partner works (unless you can and want to) or even dressing or acting a certain way. It means just being yourself and feeling good. It means embracing who you are. It means finding balance in your relationships and with the world as a whole, feeling comfortable, feeling good in your own skin, and letting other people feel good in their roles, too.

In France, where love is practically a national pastime, the heart is nourished by romantic energy. How easily the French fall in love! But in Italy, Spain, and Greece, passion is just as intense, emotions just as free, love just as ubiquitous. There is something to be said for filling up on love instead of food. Engage your passions. Reach out and touch the object of your desire (within legal limits, of course!). Love and be loved, and overeating will be the last thing on your mind.

People in the Mediterranean spend a lot of time walking, working, and just existing outside in the fresh air and sunshine. They build up the heart's endurance with hard work and fill the blood with oxygen by deeply breathing the unpolluted sea air.

Do you see how this all fits together, putting food in its place as just one part of a pleasurable life? It is all about balance. A balanced life builds a healthy heart. We can learn a lot from this approach to life. If we nourish our heart with heart-healthy food, keep our heart in good shape with exercise, fill our heart with love, and give that love away easily and openly, we can share in the spirit of the Mediterranean culture. Mediterranean-inspired pleasures are good for the heart: an appreciation for beauty, art, nature, and close friendships. The world has much to offer the seeker of pleasure, and only one slice of it has to do with food. Of course, that one slice is important to people in the Mediterranean, to me, and I'm sure to you, too.

● ●

JESSIE'S JOY

Jessie came to the United States by boat from Sicily in 1914 with her mother, Vennera, and her four brothers and sisters; Jessie was just five years old. Reunited with her father, Jessie and the family settled in Baltimore. Like so many European immigrants, Jessie and her family learned to love this country and warmly embrace American values such as freedom and opportunity. "America is a great country that opens its arms to everyone. It did for me," Jessie loved to say, and she meant every word. But, like so many first-generation immigrant families, Jessie's family brought with them the traditions and values of the "old country." Jessie grew up in the best of both cultural traditions—old and new.

Well into her eighties, Jessie still insisted on shopping at the best markets and buying only the freshest meats and produce. In the days when American moms were heartily endorsing supermarket conveniences, Jessie stubbornly chose to be "old-fashioned"; she picked out her own meats and watched the butcher cut and prepare her selections—trimming the fat and grinding hamburger from good steak. "Never buy hamburger already ground," she'd advise. Jessie rarely cooked with canned or frozen vegetables—only fresh would do.

Jessie passed away in 2003 at age ninety-four. Her granddaughter, Lee Ann, takes heart from her example. Lee Ann spent many years as an editor in New York City; now she lives in the Pacific Northwest and is our book producer, creative director of Amaranth. Lee Ann remembers trips to the markets with Jessie. She decided early on to take advantage of New York's wonderful ethnic markets and specialty grocers. Lee Ann loved talking to Jessie about Zabar's and the Union Square farmers' market and the perfect cannoli from Little Italy. Now Lee Ann enjoys perfect peaches and figs from the Port Townsend farmers' market. Thanks to Jessie's wisdom, she understands the importance of good food that is grown, purchased, and prepared with love. (And she highly recommends that you try the Copper River salmon recipe later in this chapter; Copper River salmon is a Pacific Northwest regional treasure.) Jessie always told Lee Ann, "The heart knows how to love; trust it and you'll have more than gold." I couldn't say it better myself!

• •

Nurturing your own heart and the heart of your family when you cook is a real act of love. You can do this easily by incorporating a few Mediterranean staples into your diet:

Fish: The omega-3 fatty acids in fish has been proven to help lower bad cholesterol levels and increase good cholesterol to keep your heart strong and healthy. Coldwater fish such as salmon is full of omega-3s, but all wild-caught and organic fish is good for you and a source of protein and other nutrients. I always choose wild-caught or organically farmed fish not only because it tastes better but because it is better for the environment. Many fish farms use steroids, coloring, and unnatural feeds to raise their fish.

Vibrantly colored fruits and vegetables: From beets and red peppers to dark leafy greens, red cabbage to tomatoes, mangoes to strawberries, fruits and vegetables with vibrant, deep, rich color contain hundreds of phytochemicals—those substances that nutritionists now believe exert powerful protective effects on the body. Phytochemicals give fruits and vegetables their colors and may boost your immune system, protect your heart, and guard against cancer. Add beauty and color to your meals while you strengthen your body's own defenses.

Chiles: Capsaicin, a component of spicy chile peppers, has several health benefits, not the least of which is its antiinflammatory properties. Studies show that inflammation is related to heart disease. Capsaicin may help protect the body against inflammation and the heart against future trouble.

Spices: Many different spices, from ginger and cinnamon to turmeric and paprika, contain antioxidants, antibacterial properties, antiinflammatory substances, and hundreds of phytochemicals that could protect your body in many ways nutritionists are only beginning to understand, from lowering cholesterol to boosting the power of your immune system.

Garlic: Research suggests that garlic may help lower blood pressure and cholesterol, both heart-protective effects. It may also boost your immune system, providing antibacterial as well as anticancer benefits.

> *You change your life by changing your heart.*
> **— Anonymous**

Here are some of my favorite recipes that will nourish your heart with ingredients that have proven heart-enhancing effects, as well as recipes that fill you with comfort, calm, and pleasure—perfect for sharing with the ones you love with all *your* heart.

Fruit Chutney

Chutney is a wonderful food to incorporate into a heart-healthy diet. It is a condiment for meat, fish, and chicken, or you can use it as a topping for rice or polenta. It's even good scooped onto a thin slice of crispy bread and it tastes just great with good cheese. But chutney is more than just a condiment. It contains antioxidant-rich fruits and other healthy ingredients: lemon, ginger, chiles, vinegar, and garlic. It adds a burst of sweet-sour-hot flavor to whatever you are eating. And the flavor bursts forth so vigorously that you'll only need a little bit of whatever you put it on to feel very satisfied.

½ pound fresh fruit, peeled and
    chopped (peaches, nectarines, plums,
    pears, apples, or mangoes)
Freshly squeezed juice of
    1 lemon
1 ounce ginger, peeled and minced
3 dried red chiles, stemmed and ground
    with a mortar and pestle (or
    substitute 2 teaspoons crushed red
    pepper flakes)

1 cup cider vinegar
1 tablespoon salt
1 tablespoon mustard seeds
4 ounces raisins
1–2 garlic cloves, peeled and minced

1. Combine all the ingredients except the garlic in a bowl.

2. Add the garlic, a little at a time, tasting as you go. You don't want the garlic to overwhelm the other flavors, so try to add just enough to get a nice balance.

3. Cover and let the flavors blend for at least 2 hours, preferably overnight. Store covered in the refrigerator for up to 1 week.

Peach-Fig Chutney

Serves 6

This chutney is perfect at the peak of summer when peaches and hot peppers are at their ripest. You can buy tamarind paste in gourmet food stores or online. Use fresh or dried figs for this recipe, and locally produced honey, if possible. Serve this chutney with chicken, fish, or even on crispy bread.

2 pounds peaches, pitted and cut into chunks

2 teaspoons freshly squeezed lime juice

1 pound figs, pitted and quartered

1½ cups cider vinegar

½ cup honey

3 teaspoons mustard seeds

3 tablespoons minced garlic

Salt to taste

2 tablespoons plus 2 teaspoons tamarind paste

2 tablespoons cored and seeded finely diced jalapeño

Put everything into a large saucepan over high heat and bring it to a boil. Reduce the heat and simmer approximately 15 minutes, or until the fruit is tender.

Mark Miller's Banana Salsa

My friend Mark Miller cooks fantastic southwestern cuisine at his Coyote Café in Santa Fe, New Mexico. He also writes wonderful cookbooks. This is his banana salsa recipe, which I love to pair with spicy foods. It isn't Mediterranean per se, but if you live in the Southwest, this recipe will be in line with the idea of eating regionally. If you grow your own peppers and herbs, even your own bananas, it doesn't matter where you live—this dish will be "local." Serve it with grilled fish, chicken, or even tortilla chips!

4 ripe bananas, cut into
    1/4-inch dice
2 teaspoons cored, seeded, and minced
    serrano chiles
2 teaspoons corn oil or palm oil
2 tablespoons freshly squeezed lime
    juice

2 tablespoons minced fresh cilantro
2 teaspoons minced fresh mint
2 tablespoons tamarind paste
1/2 cup cored and seeded red bell pepper
    cut into 1/4-inch dice

Mix all ingredients together and chill, covered, for at least 1 hour. Serve cold.

Heirloom Brandywine Tomato Gazpacho

Serves 4

Gazpacho is the ideal summer soup, served cold and brimming with fresh vegetables. What could be better for your heart or your soul on a sultry day? This recipe can use up your summer tomatoes that are a little past ripe or that don't look quite pretty and perfect enough for slicing. Or, buy those seconds or "uglies" at the farmers' market. Nobody will ever know those tasty tomatoes were less than perfect. If you can't find heirloom Brandywine tomatoes, any fresh, ripe local varieties will work fine. Garnish this soup with the brunoise recipe following this one. Brunoise is a mixture of fresh vegetables chopped into very small dice and used as a garnish for soup or sauce. This one adds texture and extra flavor to the gazpacho.

1 pound Heirloom Brandywine tomatoes (the softer the better), cored, seeded, and chopped

1/2 medium red onion, peeled and chopped

1/2 cup bread cubes (preferably levain sourdough with crust removed)

1 roasted poblano chile, peeled, seeded, and chopped (see page 67)

1 serrano chile, seeded and chopped

1/4 teaspoon cumin

1/4 teaspoon coriander

1/4 teaspoon smoked paprika

2 tablespoons chopped fresh cilantro

1 tablespoon chopped fresh oregano

2 tablespoons sherry vinegar

1 cup tomato juice

1/2 teaspoon minced garlic

Extra-virgin olive oil to taste

Salt and freshly ground black pepper to taste

Brunoise (recipe follows)

1 bunch scallions, sliced on bias, for garnish

1. Combine the tomatoes, onions, bread cubes, chiles, cumin, coriander, paprika, cilantro, oregano, vinegar, tomato juice, and garlic in a bowl. Cover the bowl and refrigerate overnight.

2. Put the tomato mixture through the medium dice on a food mill or process by pulsing in a food processor.

3. Stir in the olive oil. Add salt and pepper to taste.

4. Stir in the brunoise right before serving.

5. Ladle the soup into bowls and top with the scallions.

Brunoise

Use this brunoise to garnish the gazpacho or any fresh soup. You can also sprinkle it over roasted vegetables or fish. Traditionally, the vegetables for the brunoise are chopped immediately before serving for the freshest possible taste.

1 red bell pepper, cored, seeded, and diced

1 yellow bell pepper, cored, seeded, and diced

½ European cucumber, diced

1 medium red onion, peeled and diced

¼ cup chopped fresh cilantro

Combine all the ingredients in a small bowl right before serving.

Eggplant Escalivada

Serves 6 to 8 as a side dish

Escalivada actually means "cooked in the coals." If you have a grill, you can do it the old way. If not, you can roast the vegetables in a hot oven. This is great as a meze or as part of an antipasto, or served with grilled chicken or fish.

2 large eggplant	1/2 cup sherry vinegar
4 red bell peppers	1/4 cup red wine vinegar
2 tablespoons extra-virgin olive oil	1 tablespoon chopped fresh oregano
2 medium onions, peeled and sliced	Salt and pepper to taste
3 garlic cloves, peeled and thinly sliced	

1. Preheat the oven to 400°F. Rub the eggplant and the peppers with 1 tablespoon of the olive oil and roast in a roasting pan for 30 minutes until they are soft, then place them immediately in a bowl and cover with plastic wrap. Let them steam for 15 minutes. Peel them and cut them into strips. Set aside.

2. Meanwhile, heat the remaining 1 tablespoon olive oil in a medium sauté pan over medium-high heat. Add the onions and garlic and cook, stirring, until translucent, about 5 minutes. Add the vinegars and bring the mixture to a boil.

3. Pour the onion mixture over the eggplant and peppers. Mix in the oregano and salt and pepper. Serve hot or cold.

Braised Red Cabbage

Red cabbage is a great source of vitamin C and fiber, both very good for your heart. This recipe is easy. It makes an excellent holiday side dish, but it is also good for every day. Try it with lean pork or a tender piece of lamb and mashed potatoes.

2 tablespoons unsalted butter

2 tablespoons extra-virgin olive oil

2 small onions, peeled and sliced

2 garlic cloves, peeled and minced

2 apples (preferably Granny Smith),
    cored, peeled, and sliced

1/8 teaspoon ground cloves

1/8 teaspoon ground cinnamon

1/8 teaspoon ground allspice

2 bay leaves

3 tablespoons currant jelly

1 1/2 cups red wine vinegar

1 cup apple cider

1 small head red cabbage, shredded

2 tablespoons cornstarch

3 tablespoons cold water

Salt and pepper to taste

1. Heat a large stockpot over medium heat. Add the butter and olive oil. Let them foam, then add the onions and cook until they are translucent, 3–4 minutes.

2. Add the garlic and sauté 2 more minutes. Add the apples, cloves, cinnamon, allspice, and bay leaves and sauté 3 more minutes. Add the currant jelly, vinegar, and cider, and turn the heat to high, bringing to a boil.

3. When boiling, add the cabbage and stir well. Turn the heat back down to medium and cook until the cabbage is softened, 15–20 minutes.

4. Stir the cornstarch and water together in a bowl. Add the cornstarch mixture to the cabbage and combine thoroughly. Add salt and pepper to taste. Serve hot.

Orange-Dusted Seared Copper River Salmon

with Beet Salad, Blood Orange Vinaigrette,

and Baby Beet Greens

Serves 4

This recipe features salmon, which we've long known is one of the best foods you can eat for a healthy heart. Dusted with orange and surrounded by deeply colored, rich tasting beets, beet greens, and blood orange vinaigrette, this delicious recipe is like a gift to your heart. Serving it is a gift to your family, too.

3 organic blood oranges

1 cup sugar

1 cup plus 3 tablespoons water

2 shallots, peeled and minced

2 large beets, roasted in a 400°F oven
   for 30 minutes, then peeled and
   diced small

3 tablespoons red wine vinegar

Salt and pepper to taste

1/2 cup orange oil (Agrumato is best)

1 tablespoon extra-virgin olive oil

1 pound salmon fillet, preferably wild
   Alaskan or Copper River

1 tablespoon unsalted butter

2 pints baby beet greens

1. Cut just the very outer zest from two of the oranges and set it aside. Squeeze the juice from the two peeled oranges and set that aside.

2. In a medium saucepan, bring the sugar and 1 cup water to a boil over high heat. Add the orange zest and cook 10–15 minutes.

3. Preheat the oven to 250°F. Pour the sugar water with orange zest onto a baking sheet lined with parchment paper. Turn off the oven and put it in the oven to dry. This takes about 2 hours

if you have a pilot light, but ovens vary, so it could take up to 4 hours. The sugar water should be dry, not pliable, but not browned. When the mixture has dried, puree it to a fine dust in a spice grinder or blender. Set aside.

4. Place the shallots in a bowl with 1 tablespoon diced beets, the reserved orange juice, a pinch of the orange dust, the vinegar, salt, and pepper. Let it sit 10–15 minutes, then whisk in the orange oil. Taste and add more salt and pepper if necessary. Set the vinaigrette aside.

5. Put the butter and remaining 3 tablespoons water in a saucepan, and add the remaining beets. Heat over medium-high until the beets are glazed, about 8 minutes. Season with salt and pepper.

6. Meanwhile, heat a large skillet over high heat and add the olive oil. Season the salmon with salt, pepper, and orange dust. Sear in the hot olive oil, caramelizing on all sides, about 5 minutes.

7. Peel and slice the remaining orange and arrange the slices on a platter. Spoon the glazed beets onto one side of the platter and place the seared salmon beside them.

8. Toss the baby beet greens in the vinaigrette and pile on top of the salmon and beets. Drizzle the remaining vinaigrette over the platter. Serve warm.

Crab with Charred Heirloom Tomatoes and Arugula

Serves 4

This salad combines lycopene-rich tomatoes and nutrient-dense arugula with fresh crab for a lighthearted lunch.

1 pound Maine Jonah crabmeat (or use a good-quality canned crabmeat if you can't get fresh)

1 bunch scallions (about 5 scallions), white and green parts, chopped

1 jalapeño, cored, seeded, and minced (leave some seeds for spicier taste)

Salt and pepper to taste

2 tablespoons extra-virgin olive oil

2 tablespoons virgin or refined olive oil

1 pound Heirloom tomatoes (or any fresh vine-ripened tomatoes)

1 bunch arugula

1. In a medium bowl, combine the crabmeat, scallions, jalapeños, salt, and pepper. Add the extra-virgin olive oil and stir. Set aside.

2. Heat a cast iron or other heavy skillet over medium-high heat. Add the virgin or refined olive oil to the skillet and let it smoke.

3. Meanwhile, slice the tomatoes into 1-inch-thick slices, and season with salt and pepper.

4. Sear each tomato in the hot oil, being careful not to char too much. Remove the tomatoes from the skillet and chop them.

5. Divide the arugula between four salad plates, setting aside a little for garnishing. Place a spoonful of crab salad onto each pile of arugula, then top with the charred tomatoes and garnish with additional arugula. Serve immediately.

Strawberry Rhubarb Compote

This is like a strawberry-rhubarb pie without the crust. It is sweet, tart, and so delicious that it will do your heart good to eat it for dessert when strawberries and rhubarb are in season in late spring. Optionally, add two sprigs of fresh lemon verbena or lemon balm to the pot after it comes to a boil for a fragrant variation.

1 pint fresh strawberries, hulled and cut into quarters

3 stalks rhubarb, chopped

2 cups sugar

1 vanilla bean, split lengthwise and scraped

1 tablespoon freshly squeezed lemon juice

1. Place all the ingredients in a stainless steel or nonstick pot (not aluminum or cast iron) and place over medium-high heat.

2. Bring the mixture to a boil, stirring occasionally, then turn down to a simmer and cook just until the rhubarb begins to break down, about 15 minutes. Remove the vanilla bean. Serve warm or chilled.

What I'd like you to take away from this chapter is simple: Keep your heart healthy by moving a lot, loving a lot, and eating heart-protective foods such as fish, fresh fruits and vegetables, and olive oil. And don't forget to keep your heart open to others. Love is the best exercise of all for that beautiful heart beating inside you.

13

Nothing New Under the Sun

If you lived in the Mediterranean in some little town along the coastline, you would probably spend much of your day outside. You would move a lot, perhaps garden a lot, perhaps swim or climb or run. You would walk to the market, and you would walk home with your basket of food. You would cook, clean, and work. Maybe you would care for children or spend time helping friends with their work. Sometimes you would sit together with friends or family and enjoy a meal or a cup of coffee. And then you would go back to work. Chances are, you would be very healthy.

This simple Mediterranean lifestyle hasn't changed all that much over the years. You can still find little towns with one store and one tiny gathering spot for food and drink. "What do people do all day?" a friend of mine asked on a recent trip to Italy as she walked through a tiny village that didn't have television, Internet service, malls or convenience stores, movie theaters, or even very many cars. But people *were* doing things—they were walking and talking, gathering to eat together, cooking and cleaning, and spending a lot of time outside simply being where they were, their minds happily present. What a concept. Everyone seemed strong, healthy, and very relaxed.

Much of the Mediterranean way boils down to one concept: simplicity. Sometimes the old ways are the best ways. Simplicity in the form of simple food, simple exercise, and a simple life with less pressure and more basic human interaction is the hallmark of the Mediterranean way.

The Greek word for "diet" is *diata*, but a direct translation doesn't refer to mere calorie intake. It can more accurately be translated as "lifestyle." The Mediterranean "diet" isn't just an eating plan of so many calories and so much fat per day. It is a lifestyle that touches everything you do—how much physical activity you get, how strong your social connections are, how much time you take to enjoy the pleasures of life, and yes, also what you eat.

Before 1960, the people of the Mediterranean enjoyed the lowest heart disease and cancer rates and the greatest longevity of almost anywhere in the world, but then American influences began to change people's habits. So let's look back at how life was in the 1950s in the Mediterranean, when Americans were eating their three square meals of meat and potatoes each day . . . and dying young of heart attacks. While we obviously can't travel back in a time machine, fortunately we can get a glimpse of the old ways by looking at some of the smaller rural communities in the Mediterranean, which have remained largely unchanged for decades.

☀ Life Then and Now

When Price and I were bicycling all over Sicily, we felt as if we had gone back in that very time machine. Life was so much different there, the energy of the place a radical change from the energy in America, or really any larger city. It's easy to envision how life has long been for many of these people by watching them today as they balance their hard physical work with the leisure activities they so treasure, as they maintain their close-knit communities and families, and as they prepare and enjoy food together.

> *Who can ever be alone for a moment in Italy? Every stone has a voice, every grain of dust seems instinct with spirit from the Past, every step recalls some line, some legend of long-neglected lore.*

> — **Margaret Fuller, writer**

On an island such as Sicily, the land space isn't all that big, so people are automatically pushed closer together. But unlike the impression you get in a large city such as New York, people seem to enjoy this closeness. They talk freely and openly, they look each other in the eye, and they depend on each other.

In big cities, I've noticed that the closer people physically get to each other, the more they withdraw emotionally from each other. People stay inside on their computers where they don't have to interact with the crowds. When women walk down the street, their eyes are straight ahead to avoid eye contact. This isn't just American stubbornness — it can be a matter of safety.

In rural Mediterranean communities, life is much different. People greet each other with a *"Buon giorno"* or *"Ciao!"* People help each other, and many women live with several generations of their family in one home. People take over family businesses from their parents. Children grow up knowing their grandparents. Friends stay together for years. Women spend time with other women. Even when they spend time alone, it is with pleasure and inner peace.

Part of this has to do with the fact that many women in the Mediterranean stay put. Their birthplace becomes a part of who they know themselves to be. It helps to ground them with a sense of self and a sense of community.

If you live in a smaller town, you may be thinking this way of life doesn't seem so out of reach. Where I live in Maine, life is quite similar to what I saw in Sicily. People often live here for their entire lives, stay in close touch with family and friends, and maintain a slower pace of life. My point is that you don't have to go to the Mediterranean or be from the Mediterranean to achieve a greater balance between work and leisure. And you don't have to spend your entire life in your hometown to feel connected to the place in which you live. You just have to make a conscious effort to open yourself to your community, your neighbors, even your own climate. Let it become a part of who you are even if you have only lived there a short while.

If you do live in a big city, you don't have to get sucked into a high-stress, complicated lifestyle, either. You may be very busy, but you can still slow down for meals and savor every bite. You can slow down in your thinking for at least a little while every day and breathe. You can sit in an outdoor cafe and enjoy a cup of coffee before you continue with your busy day. Whenever you eat or drink anything at all, you can stop doing everything else. Just enjoy the moment.

Try sitting in a cafe for a while and see how it goes. Watch the people, but in your own body, stop! Can you stand it? Do you want to pull out your laptop and e-mail someone? Are your fingers itching to dial a friend on your cell phone? Do you feel compelled to read a magazine? Or can you just sip that coffee or tea or water with lemon and do only that? Remember, only habit keeps you from being present.

There are many ways to capture the Mediterranean spirit of simplicity. I'm not asking you to forego the pleasures and luxuries that you enjoy. *Au contraire!* I'm asking you to savor what matters. You can spend more time with friends, stay in closer touch with your family, volunteer in your community, or rent a plot in a community garden. You can stop constantly buying things for entertainment and start spending more time outside. You can do one thing at a time. Just set aside a little time for simplicity each day.

> *Italians are never punctual; the cafe, the convenient place to wait, absolves them from that. There is no question of hanging about, no looking lost and unwanted or even disreputable, as there is in hotel lobbies or the foyers of restaurants. One just sits and enjoys the scene, and waits.*
> —**Shirley Hazzard, writer**

☀ Move It or Lose It

About that walking I keep mentioning—this is another distinct difference between the lifestyles of the typical American woman and the typical woman living along the Mediterranean Sea: exercise. Life in the Mediterranean, particularly a few decades ago, was full of physical labor. Women spent a lot of time outside, working, moving, lifting, walking. They had gardens to tend, animals to feed, food to harvest. When they went to the market or to visit a friend, they walked or bicycled. Children played outside, never inside in front of a television with a video game controller in hand.

In the United States, city dwellers often walk a lot. But rural and suburban dwellers usually drive everywhere—to the store, to the neighbor's house, even to their own mailboxes! Getting outside and walking or bicycling to the places you need to go is quintessentially Mediterranean. When you walk, you get full access to the sunshine, fresh air, and direct experience of your own community. This is a natural and integral part of Mediterranean life, and it can be a natural part of your life, too. Just put down your car keys and get out there.

Think of all the ways you could rely less on technology and more on your own steam. Make bread by hand. Walk to work. Dig up that garden plot with a shovel instead of a tiller. Hand wash your dishes. Walk to the store and carry your groceries home—if you go every day, you won't have to fill up the whole grocery cart, and your food will be fresher. The next time you want to watch television, go on a bicycle ride and watch the scenery instead. Turn the compost with a pitchfork. Walk your dog. Play kickball with your kids. Go swimming. Walk home from work.

• •

LUCY'S LIFE

Primo head grower Lucy Funkhouser Yanz may be seven months pregnant, but that doesn't keep her from working in Primo's organic gardens. Every bit a twenty-first-century American woman, Lucy nevertheless leads a very traditional Mediterranean life. Her exercise plan these days consists of weeding, composting, digging, transplanting, harvesting, and contemplating in the gardens.

Lucy grew up in the Mediterranean way thanks to her mother, who always cooked in that tradition, although she was not from the Mediterranean. "Being pregnant has made me even more committed to eating healthy food," Lucy says. "I've been trying to eat a lot of protein, and I've been making a lot of frittatas using the vegetables we get from CSA [the Community-Supported Agriculture program]. My healthy habits have stuck with me, but I think it really helps how active I am." Lucy is outside most of the day gardening. "I think gardening is a really good way of keeping your body in balance. I don't feel like eating a lot because I'm working so much," explains Lucy.

Lucy came to gardening when she was eighteen. "That's when I became interested in more sustainable ways of living," says Lucy. She and her husband try to eat locally produced, seasonal food whenever possible. "We want what we eat to reflect what's going on around us. We don't buy watermelons and cucumbers out of season. It makes the different foods that much more exciting when they come into season. I've been trying to eat more and more that way, to not get impatient and buy things out of season but to wait until they come into season here."

When food does come into season, Lucy preserves it or freezes it to extend the growing season while still supporting local producers. "Eating like this is better, more frugal, and to me, it just makes more sense," says Lucy.

• •

Of course, there is nothing wrong with exercising in more formal (and more American) settings such as the gym, or in less utilitarian ways such as jogging without a destination. If that is the way you like to exercise, great! The end result is the same: you get healthier, your heart stays strong, and you feel better about yourself and your body.

A recent study showed that regular aerobic exercise was just as effective as antidepressant medication in relieving symptoms of depression. We spend so much time sitting inside at a desk, in front of a computer, on a couch in front of the television, or in our cars with the radio blaring that we lose touch with our bodies and the way they move. Find your body again and let it move. And at least every now and then, let your body move outside. You don't have to live in the Mediterranean to get back in touch with the natural world—just go outside and walk. Or just step outside for a few moments and breathe.

☀ Nature Girl

Give your body a break from stale indoor air. Open your windows in your home for at least an hour each day. Long, full, deep breathing suffuses your body with oxygen. Step outside on your breaks at work and breathe. Let Nature in.

You can also get your few minutes with Nature each day by standing barefoot in a patch of grass, letting the sun shine on your skin, even for just five or ten minutes each day, and looking at wildlife. Contemplate the way the wind moves through the tree branches. Consider how you are part of the natural world, too—not just living with it but being of it.

Nature is powerful enough to reset your internal rhythms and help you slow down, relax, breathe. This is how stress drains away, and you know what chronic stress does to you: it makes you tense, uncomfortable, and probably makes you eat more without enjoying your food.

> *My heart is like a singing bird.*
> —**Christina Rossetti, poet**

Here are some more ideas for how you can get outside, move, breathe, and let Nature into your life:

• Take a walk to new places. Discover nearby parks you've never visited. Walk slow, walk fast, but engage with the world around you as you go. Look for signs of the natural world. Birds? Clouds? Trees? Flowers?

• Get out that old bicycle and ride around your neighborhood. Explore areas you wouldn't normally have time to explore if you were walking.

• Put a basket on your bicycle and ride to the grocery store for the food you need for tonight's dinner. Think how French you'll feel, riding your bike home with a long, skinny baguette in your bicycle basket!

• Plant a garden in your yard, in containers on your deck or front porch, even in window boxes. Try tomatoes, peppers, eggplant, peas, beans, carrots, radishes, and fresh greens. What else might grow in your area? One clue is to try growing what you normally see offered at the farmers' market.

• Grow herbs. Tending a small herb garden or tea garden is an exercise in aesthetics, and the aromas you will experience every time you weed the garden or harvest the plants will help you tune in to the natural world and give your mind a break from all your other responsibilities.

• Drag your children outside. Tell them, "Step away from the video games!" Take them on day trips, such as to nearby national forests, parks, lakes, beaches, and hiking trails. If they complain, that's a sign that they are not doing this kind of thing nearly enough. In their natural environments, children are supposed to love this kind of thing! Jane Austen wrote, "They are to be pitied, who have not been . . . given a taste for nature in early life." Mediterranean children get that taste. Don't your kids deserve it, too?

• If you don't have children, take a friend who also needs to get away from her computer. Or take your dog. Or your friend and your dog! Or just go yourself if you need a break from people. Let Nature be your companion.

• Mow the lawn. Trim the bushes. Prune the trees. Weed the roses along the driveway. Tend your yard as if it were your very own country estate. Why hire a neighbor kid to have all the fun?

• The next time a friend suggests meeting for coffee, counter with a suggestion that you get your coffee to go and take a walk in the fresh air.

• On a rainy day, put on your boots and grab an umbrella. Go for a walk in the rain. Splash in the puddles. (Not sure about that? Let a kid show you how.) Or just stand outside under the cover of an eave and watch how the rain changes the world.

• Go swimming in a natural body of water—100 percent chlorine-free. Whether an ocean, a local lake, or a reservoir, feel how different it is to soak in water that is part of the earth's natural cycle. You don't have to put your head under—just let the water rock you, and let go of everything else.

• Once a week, get up, go outside, and watch the sunrise. Once a week, stop what you are doing and go outside to watch the sun set. Once a week, notice what stage the moon is in. Is it full, a tiny sliver, or halfway between the two? Look at the stars and see what the sky promises for tomorrow.

> *We are nature. We are nature seeing nature. We are nature with a concept of nature. Nature weeping. Nature speaking of nature to nature.*
>
> **—Susan Griffin, poet**

• Cultivate an interest in your local wildlife. Discover what birds are native to your area, and look for them. Or become an expert on the local wildflowers, or the food crops that grow best in your area, or wild foods. Go foraging for mushrooms, wild onions, and greens. (Be sure about what you eat—some wild mushrooms, greens, and berries are not edible.)

• Get off the asphalt. Most cities and towns have hiking trails and off-road bicycle trails you can explore through parks or other wildlife areas.

• Just once, when the weather is lovely, sleep outside in a tent, on a deck, even within a screened-in porch. In her book *A Country Year*, Sue Hubbell wrote, "I have stopped sleeping inside. A house is too small, too confining. I want the whole world, and the stars too." Take them!

• On your next vacation, choose a place where you can really get into Nature. You don't have to make this quest the entire sum of your vacation, but let it be one important part. Hike up a mountain, swim in the ocean, get totally surrounded by trees, explore a glacier. What *can't* you do at home?

These are the keys to enjoying a more Mediterranean way of life: Make a commitment to stay in touch with your family. Spend more time with your friends. Let them unburden you. Talk to them. Stay in touch. Move more. Exercise every day. Spend time each day in Nature, breathing the air, feeling the sun, working in your garden, playing with your kids in a park, going for walks. Slow down and let a little of every day be made of leisure.

And when you eat? Taste. Savor. Let your meal become the whole of your experience. That's the Mediterranean way.

Let the Mediterranean lifestyle lull you into a more stress-free, relaxed way of living. You can still get your work done, but you'll enjoy it more. You might even do a better job. This spirit can make your life more vivid and more worth living. I really believe that. Why don't you join me?

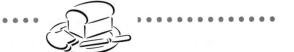

14

Artigiano

Putting all the pieces of the Mediterranean way together to create a unified vision and method for living is much like producing a work of art. Become a Mediterranean food artist and you may find yourself smiling the knowing smile of the *Mona Lisa*! Soul, heart, family, love, friendship, the earth, are all inextricably linked through food and make up the elements of the artist's palette. And the artist is you. Think of a mosaic. Each piece of brightly colored tile fits into the whole picture to create something beautiful, memorable, lasting.

But it can be hard to grasp how to put all these pieces together, especially when the Mediterranean way isn't ingrained in you from childhood the way it is for so many women who actually live there or whose parents came to America from there. How do you eat day to day? How do you know how much to put on your plate, what to choose, when to make which recipes? This chapter is here for you!

For those of you who like more exacting rules than just "eat better, eat less," the following seven-day meal planner uses the recipes in this book to give you guidance on what and how much to eat in traditional Mediterranean fashion. Each day includes breakfast, lunch, an afternoon taste, dinner, and an evening taste. Each is portion controlled and contains wholesome plant foods with just a little meat here and there for excitement. Take a little time to cook with care each day, to prepare your food lovingly, and to eat slowly, savoring every bite, and I think you'll find this week of eating very pleasurable. Use this meal planner as a guide for creating more and more weeks of Mediterranean eating in the same style and spirit. If you enjoy having your meals mapped out for you, check out ediets.com. This service helps you track your weight loss, hook up with support groups, and custom-designs menus and shopping lists for you, all online. Their newest meal-plan option: The Mediterranean Diet!

Sunday

Sunday is a good day to have a nice family meal together for dinner. You may also have more time to cook on Sunday, so some of these meals take a little more preparation time than meals during the week.

Breakfast

2 eggs, scrambled, topped with ¼ cup Salsa Verde (page 45)

1 slice rye bread, toasted, drizzled with 1 teaspoon olive oil

1 small orange

Lunch
>   1 serving Bread and Fish Soup (page 65)
>   1 cup steamed snow peas
>   1 cup red grapes

Afternoon Taste
>   1 cup sliced strawberries mixed with 1 ounce goat
>   cheese and 1 tablespoon slivered almonds

Dinner
>   1 serving Grilled Tenderloin of Beef with Iowa Blue
>   Cheese Potato Gratin, Caramelized Cipollini Onions,
>   and Porcini Mushrooms (page 156)
>   2 cups salad greens with Balsamic Vinaigrette
>   (page 88)
>   1 cup cubed honeydew melon

Evening Taste
>   ¼ cup low-fat cottage cheese
>   ½ cup raspberries
>   8 unsalted peanuts

Monday

The work week begins. Who has time to cook? Today's menu is
quick and easy.

Breakfast
>   2 slices whole-wheat toast spread with 1 tablespoon
>   organic peanut butter
>   2 cups cubed cantaloupe
>   1 ounce mozzarella cheese

Lunch

  2 cups Cherry Tomato Salad (page 104)

  ½ of 6-inch whole-wheat pita or *piadina*

  3 ounces tuna packed in water or olive oil mixed with
     ½ cup Pepperonata all'Abruzzese (page 59; prepared
     ahead)

Afternoon Taste

  1 cup plain yogurt mixed with ¾ cup blueberries,
     1 tablespoon wheat germ, and 1 teaspoon honey

Dinner

  1 serving Pasta Alla Puttanesca (page 187)

  1 cup steamed broccoli tossed with 1 tablespoon freshly
     grated Parmesan or pecorino cheese and 8 raw
     almonds

  1 cup chopped apples mixed with 1 tablespoon raisins
     and 1 tablespoon Candied Pecans (page 226)

Evening Taste

  6 Greek olives

  ½ cup white beans, rinsed and drained

  Lemon herbal tea

Tuesday

Now that the week is in full swing, don't forget to eat well.

Breakfast
>   1 serving Farmer's Omelet (page 105)
>   1 slice rye bread, toasted, drizzled with 1 teaspoon
>   olive oil
>   ½ grapefruit

Lunch
>   1 slice toasted whole-wheat bread topped with ¼ cup
>   Caponata (page 70)
>   ¾ cup raspberries
>   ½ cup plain yogurt
>   1 tablespoon cashews

Afternoon Taste
>   1 ounce tuna packed in water or olive oil mixed with
>   1 stalk celery, diced, and ½ cup grapes, cut in half

Dinner
>   Antipasto Platter containing the following:
>   Assorted cut raw vegetables with Bagna Cauda
>   (page 85)
>   1 serving Field Greens with Roasted Beets and Fresh
>   Sheep's Cheese (page 71)
>   ¼ toasted whole-wheat pita topped with 1 tablespoon
>   Caponata (page 70)
>   1 serving Tuna with Cabernet Whipped Potatoes
>   (page 215)
>   1½ cups cubed honeydew melon

Evening Taste
   ¼ toasted whole-wheat pita spread with 1 tablespoon
      goat cheese and 1 tablespoon chopped Greek olives

Wednesday

....

Don't forget to stay in touch with your family today. Can you all
sit down for dinner at the same time? Sure you can!

Breakfast
   1 cup low-fat cottage cheese mixed with ½ cup
      blueberries, ½ cup sliced strawberries, ½ cup
      raspberries, and 2 tablespoons slivered almonds

Lunch
   1 serving Vegetable Terrine (page 109)
   4 ounces plain yogurt mixed with 1 tablespoon
      walnuts
   1 Granny Smith apple

Afternoon Taste
   ½ of 6-inch whole-wheat pita, toasted and topped with
      1 tablespoon tomato sauce, dash of oregano, and
      1 ounce shredded mozzarella cheese, baked until
      cheese is melted

Dinner
   1 serving Quick-Cooked Salmon with Fall Vegetable
      Pistou (page 171)
   1 serving Curried Couscous Pilaf (page 142)
   2 cups raw baby spinach topped with 1 tablespoon

Balsamic Vinaigrette (page 88)
1 cup sliced strawberries

Evening Taste
1 stalk celery, chopped, combined with 1 small chopped
apple, 2 tablespoons plain yogurt, and 1 tablespoon
raisins

Thursday

Today, try a change of scenery. Can you eat dinner outside in
the fresh air or at least in front of a big window?

Breakfast
½ of 6-inch whole-wheat pita, toasted, stuffed with
1 sliced tomato, 2 ounces mozzarella cheese, ¼ cup
white beans, and 1 tablespoon chopped fresh basil

Lunch
Assorted cut raw vegetables with Bagna Cauda
(page 85)
3 ounces grilled or broiled chicken breast mixed with
¼ cup garbanzo beans, 1 hard-boiled egg, chopped,
¼ cup chopped green onions, and 1 tablespoon
Balsamic Vinaigrette (page 88)
1 cup cubed cantaloupe

Afternoon Taste
1 cup popcorn sprinkled with ½ teaspoon garlic powder
and 1 tablespoon grated Parmesan cheese

Dinner
   1 serving Farro Ragout (page 148)
   1 serving Parsnip Mashed Potatoes (page 191)
   2 cups Lucy's Salad (page 68) topped with 2 ounces
      fresh sheep's cheese

Evening Taste
   2 ounces Sean Kelly's Rosemary Roasted Almonds
      (page 180)

Friday

The weekend is practically here. Have you planned some leisure time?

Breakfast
   1 cup plain yogurt layered with 1 tablespoon wheat germ,
      ½ cup blueberries, and 1 tablespoon chopped walnuts

Lunch
   1 serving Yellow Velvet Soup (page 186)
   1 tomato, cored and stuffed with 3 ounces salmon (fresh
      or canned)
   6 baby carrots
   1 cup green grapes

Afternoon Taste
   1 hard-boiled egg, chopped, mixed with 1 stalk celery,
      chopped, 1 minced garlic clove, 2 tablespoons
      plain yogurt, and 1 teaspoon freshly squeezed
      lemon juice

Dinner

> 1 serving Pasta with Tomato-Pepper Coulis (page 231)
> 1 serving Artichokes with Lemon Aioli (page 183)
> 1 serving Fresh Corn Fritters (page 232)
> 2 cups mixed baby greens with 2 teaspoons olive oil and
> 1 tablespoon freshly squeezed lemon juice

Evening Taste

> ½ cup garbanzo beans topped with 2 tablespoons Mint
> Yogurt (page 43)

Saturday

The weekend is a nice time to enjoy dessert with dinner. Savor a small piece of cheesecake and enjoy every bite.

Breakfast

> 1 serving Fresh Sheep's Ricotta Frittata with
> Mushrooms and Herbs (page 229)
> 1 cup sliced strawberries

Lunch

> 1 serving Prosciutto, Fennel, and Pear Salad with
> Persimmon Vinaigrette (page 129)
> 1 serving Pissaladière (page 74)
> 1 orange

Afternoon Taste

> 1 baguette slice spread with 1 tablespoon Tapenade
> (page 37)

Dinner
> 1 serving Heirloom Brandywine Tomato Gazpacho
> (page 245)
> 1 serving Charred Lamb Salad (page 153)
> 1 serving Wild Mushroom Risotto (page 146)
> 1 serving Ricotta Cheesecake (page 233)

Evening Taste
> ½ cup applesauce mixed with 1 tablespoon walnuts
> 1 ounce mozzarella cheese

Of course, food isn't the only piece of Mediterranean life that you can incorporate into your own life for better health, a better body, and a happier, freer, more passionate approach to living.

✳ Finding Your Natural Balance

Living in the spirit of the Mediterranean takes balance. This is sometimes hard for American women to grasp because we tend to do everything to the extreme—total absorption or total deprivation. It isn't easy, either, to step back and really look at your life and how balanced or imbalanced it is. Do you feel good? Do you love the way you feel? Do you feel in touch with your feminine self, or are you too busy running everything?

Nobody feels balanced all the time, but if you feel like you are living on the edge of a cliff, just barely holding it together from day to day, or even if you feel that you aren't quite fulfilled, spend some time in self-reflection. What if you lived by the sea and could smell it, see it, and listen to the waves on the shore every single day? What if you could just let your free, vital, open nature go? What if you loved your best features and didn't worry about the others? What if your approach to life was breezy, frank, and one moment at a time?

Also consider how different your life might be if your parents lived in your home, and your children and your grandparents, too, and (this may be the hard part to imagine) everyone *loved* it that way? What if your friends came over to talk with you every day or met you in the market and you picked out the day's menus together? What if everywhere you went, you felt the influence of sun and salt, olive trees and fresh fish, fruits and vegetables bursting and ripe? What if you never had to go into a supermarket, a mall, a convenience store, or a giant discount warehouse ever again? What if you never even knew what those things were?

What if you had enough time? What if everywhere you went, you felt absolutely gorgeous? What if you loved every inch of yourself? What kind of artistic masterpiece would your life be then? It would be yours—handcrafted and unique.

> *Women need real moments of solitude and self-reflection to balance out how much of ourselves we give away.*
>
> **—Barbara De Angelis, writer**

I'm not trying to get you to feel dissatisfied with your life, not one bit. I would just like you to think about what is going on in your life. Think about the parts you love and the parts you wish worked better. Assuming you aren't going to pick up and move to Sicily, Greece, Spain, or southern France, how could the principles of living in the Mediterranean style and spirit help guide you toward greater balance, satisfaction, and happiness? How can you take the Mediterranean woman's approach to life and incorporate it into your own? What parts can you take from that ancient wisdom, and what parts of your life do you cherish and want to keep? Ask yourself these questions:

- Do I take enough time to relax every day?

- Do I feel healthy most of the time?

- Do I like the way I look? Do I wish I weighed less or more?

- Do I feel strong?

- Do I feel self-confident? Do I like the kind of person I have become? Do I like who I am right now, today?

- When did I last spend time outside noticing the world?

- Do I have a place to go where the air is fresh and I can see signs of nature thriving? How often do I go there?

- Do I spend enough time with my children? Would they say I do?

- Does my family sit down together for dinner at least once every week? Do we talk and enjoy each other?

- Do I know how to process negative emotions, let go of them, and move on? Or are they stuck inside me?

- Do I spend enough time with my spouse/partner? Do I really focus on that person or am I usually distracted? What would my spouse/partner say about this?

- Do I get enough exercise to feel comfortable in my body? Do I move vigorously for at least twenty minutes every day?

- Do I feel satisfied with the work I do? Is it worthwhile? Is it fulfilling? Am I living my dream?

- What is my dream? Is it realistic? Can I make it happen? What am I doing to move toward that dream?

- Do I take a vacation every year? Do I actually go somewhere? Do I enjoy it?

- How much time do I spend every day staring at some kind of screen? Sitting in a chair?

- Are my relationships with my friends rewarding to me? Do I have enough social contact with friends?

- Do I know how to share my feelings with my friends? Do they know how to help me process those feelings?

- Do I know how to listen to my friends? Do I know how to help them when they need help? Do I choose to help them?

- Do I know how to say no when people are making too many demands on my time?

- How often do I talk with my relatives? Do I wish it was more or less?

- Do I feel connected to my family, or my spouse's family, or any family?

- How often do I touch someone passionately? How much affection do I get? Is it enough?

- How much of myself do I offer to my community? Do I feel that I should be volunteering more of my time or resources to others in need?

- What was the last thing I gave to someone else?

- What the heck have I been eating lately?

Chances are, your answers to some of these questions aren't what you wish they were. Make a list of those things you would like to see become more balanced in your life. Attach it to the refrigerator or some other highly visible place in your home. Think about it. Mull it over. Start taking steps to bring yourself more into balance, to create the kind of life you want to be living. This is a slow process of self-discovery for some, but it is something other cultures do automatically. In our rush, our business, our obsession with time, money, success, and accomplishment, sometimes we forget.

Figuring out how to put all these elements together is largely an individual matter to work through each day in our own way. But I can give you one piece of advice about the creation of this sort of art, one tangible thing you can do to make it all come together for a little while in a way that is beautiful, satisfying, and grounded in the Mediterranean spirit: host a celebratory dinner.

> *I feel now that gastronomical perfection can be reached in these combinations: one person dining alone, usually upon a couch or a hill side; two people, of no matter what sex or age, dining in a good restaurant; six people, of no matter what sex or age, dining in a good home.*
>
> —M. F. K. Fisher, writer

Some people are very nervous about entertaining others in their homes. But it needn't be a complicated undertaking at all. When you serve a multicourse meal to others, you throw yourself into the community as someone giving to others. You create an event that will come back to you in equal measure. Offering food to others in your own home nudges you into a way of life that involves give and take. It banishes isolation. It is reaching out a hand to your friends. I'm not saying you should invite the whole city to your dinner party. Six people is just fine to start.

You will be preparing food with heart and offering it to others. This is a wonderful gesture and an act of love.

A dinner party isn't the time for fancy cutting-edge productions, however. You aren't playing chef in a fancy restaurant, after all. You want to enjoy yourself, too. I always advise making something easy that you know tastes good. This isn't the time to try something new and fancy. Stick with the tried-and-true dishes you know you make well. Here are some other things to remember when serving others in your home:

• For an interesting evening, invite a mixture of people: young and old, male and female, from different walks of life. If everybody is from the same place and doing the same thing, they will probably "talk shop," although that can be fun, too.

• Let people help you. You don't have to do it all alone. That's not in the Mediterranean spirit. Let people come into your kitchen and give them jobs to do. It will make the whole preparation experience happier and more fun.

• Prepare as much as possible ahead of time so that you can assemble courses quickly and easily.

• Let your children act as servers. Offer to pay them! Train them on what to do, but don't worry if they don't do everything perfectly. That will be part of the charm of the whole affair.

• Let yourself be whimsical. Decorate the table and the dining room (or wherever you are eating) according to the menu. Whimsy can be much more fun and relaxing than elegance.

• Flowers from your own garden or yard are more personal than a fancy arrangement from a florist.

• Candles are inexpensive and add a relaxing but mystical mood, signaling everyone that the evening is something special.

- Offer an *aperitivo*, wine with each course, and a *digestivo* to help put everyone in the frame of mind for warm socializing, and of course, for proper digestion! See chapter 10 for ideas. Don't forget nonalcoholic options.

- Don't feel compelled to clean up while guests are still in your home. You should enjoy yourself, too.

But what about the menu? If you aren't sure what to serve, try the menus here using recipes from this book. But certainly adapt these to your own needs, feelings, preferences, and of course, whatever is fresh and seasonal at the moment.

Eating is never so simple as hunger.
—**Erica Jong, writer**

Menu 1: Extended Family Meal, Italian Style

Antipasto including
    Caponata
    Fava and Pecorino Bruschetta
    Tapenade on Crostini
Pasta Alla Puttanesca
Atlantic Salmon and Green Garlic
Tuscan Bread Salad
Chocolate Gelato with Hazelnut Biscotti
Espresso

Menu 2: Spanish Tapas

Rosemary Roasted Almonds
Eggplant Escalivada
Spanish ham slices (purchased)
Crusty bread (purchased)
Salsa Verde
Merguez
Heirloom Brandywine Tomato Gazpacho
Crema Catalana

Menu 3: French Feast, à la Provencal

Pissaladière
Bread and Fish Soup
Vegetable Terrine
Quick-Cooked Salmon with Fall Vegetable Pistou
Cookies
  Langues de Chat
  Lavender Shortbread
  French Almond Wafers
  Socca
Coffee or Tisane

Meal 5: Middle Eastern Meal

Hummus and Toasted Pita
Tabbouleh Salad
Mint Yogurt
Munchkin Pumpkins with Shrimp and Couscous
Charred Lamb Salad
Baklava (purchased)
Lydia's Lebanese Coffee

Menu 6: Farmers' Market Summer Supper

Farmer's Omelet
Yellow Velvet Soup
Corn Fritters
Field Greens with Roasted Beets and Fresh Sheep's
    Cheese
Garden Strawberries with Fresh Sheep's Cheese and
    Balsamic Syrup

And how was the party? Spectacular and unique, I'm sure. As you continue to fit all the pieces together, sculpting your life into a beautiful work of art inspired by the Mediterranean but uniquely you, keep taking pleasure in your life, your food, and your own true self. That's how those women do it, you know. And that's how you can do it, too.

15

Baklava and Biscotti

How could we finish without a little something sweet? In the Mediterranean, dessert isn't a daily affair. Sweets are something special to be savored and fully experienced. The notion of getting a candy bar out of a vending machine every afternoon would seem strange and foreign to Mediterranean women. Dessert isn't meant to be convenient. It is for celebration, and it should taste very fresh and very good.

More often than not, fresh, luscious fruit ends a meal with a sweet taste but without added sugar, and this is in itself an artful dessert. Fresh fruit in season bursts with sweetness and signals the body that the meal is ending. It also makes a perfect snack between meals when hunger strikes—a juicy apple, a succulent orange, a sensual pear, a warm peach, a sunset-orange nectarine, a handful of beautiful grapes misted with that bloom that signals their absolute freshness. Whatever fruit is in season right now is what you should be eating with joy.

Deep from her blue apron pocket
she drew a ripe orange to slice
and squirt light
—your mouth was stained with sun.

— **Janet Frame, writer**

Sometimes, something baked, something frozen and creamy, or something custardy and sweet is the right choice for a special dessert. Although women do make their own desserts at home, a common Mediterranean practice is to get dessert, as well as bread, from the local baker. These desserts and breads are made fresh every day, and because home cooking is focused more on what can be done with the fresh produce from the market, the baking is left to the professionals. Some Mediterranean favorites such as baklava are just too time-consuming to make at home on a regular basis, and they are easy to buy from a good bakery. Bring home a fresh-baked pastry for your family to enjoy after dinner. If you trust your baker, you know it will be delicious. No effort or dirty dishes required.

Speaking of that afternoon vending machine run so familiar to corporate America . . . well, a midafternoon pastry is a tradition in the Mediterranean. Midafternoon is the time to find a friend, stroll into a cafe, sit, relax, savor a cup of coffee, and split a really good pastry or indulge in a small bit of really good chocolate. There is nothing hurried about it! And there is no point in eating anything sweet unless you are going to let yourself sink fully into the deep, soul-satisfying pleasure of it. This is a time to relax, contemplate your day, talk with your friends, share your stories, laugh, enjoy your warm coffee or tea, and take just a few bites of something luscious.

Chocolate is no ordinary food. It is not something
you can take or leave, something you like only

moderately. You don't like chocolate. You don't even love chocolate. Chocolate is something you have an affair with.

—Geneen Roth, writer

You don't have to walk out on your boss and defiantly go in search of a cafe. But you can stop what you are doing for fifteen minutes. You can eat something you brought from home or from somewhere that doesn't require you to insert pocket change into a slot. And you can pay attention to what you are eating. If possible, leave your desk. Go outside. Sip a warm drink. Notice every bite of your afternoon snack, no matter what it is. Look around you. Soak up the sun. Chat with a friend about something other than work. This is what taking a *break* really is, and it is something people in the Mediterranean know how to do very well. Isn't it time you practiced?

I hope you will accept that you can eat dessert if you really want to eat dessert and if the dessert is something really worth eating. But remember portion control. Moderation. The three-bite rule! A few bites of an amazing dessert or tasty sweet snack is all it takes to feel satisfied. Eating beyond those first few perfect tastes isn't really about eating for hunger or pleasure, anyway. It's usually about habit or because the food is there, or to fill an emotional void. If you are really ravenous in the mid-afternoon, you probably didn't have enough lunch. If you are still that hungry after dinner, well, perhaps you needed a bit more dinner. Have a salad to wind down the meal, as they often do in the Mediterranean.

I encourage you to find a good local baker. Price does all our baking at Primo, and people know they can get delicious fresh breads and fantastic sweet desserts made with attention and affection from Primo. Most cities have a good baker. If you find one, then all your baking needs will be met! That being said, some people really enjoy baking (just ask Price, who loves to bake even though he rarely eats sweets because he says they put him right to sleep!). For those of you who want to prepare delicious desserts for your family on special occasions, here are some of Price's favorite Mediterranean-inspired recipes.

☀ Cookies

Cookies are a wonderful way to enjoy dessert because they are preformed into a single serving size for you. Just eat one and enjoy it. And then stop. In the Mediterranean, crispy cookies are the norm, rather than the soft, gooey American variety. Keep them in an airtight container and you'll have the resources to turn your nose up at those grocery store, prepackaged, preservative-laden cookies. This is the real thing.

These cookie recipes all require the use of either a Silpat mat or parchment paper on a baking sheet. When I say Silpat, I mean either those silicone baking mats that are entirely nonstick and perfect for delicate cookies or those baking sheets made entirely of silicone. Or buy a roll of parchment paper and cut it to fit your baking sheets. The silicone baking mats are very nice to have, so you might consider investing in one if you bake often.

• •

EVE'S STORY

Eve is this book's co-author and she has been writing about the Mediterranean diet for several years now. She loves the idea of the Mediterranean diet, but in her life as a freelance food writer and single mom of two little boys, sometimes she slips into some bad dietary habits. "I write about food all the time, but I have very little time to actually cook it! Or, at least, I tell myself I don't have enough time, and that's when I pick up the phone and order a pizza. But when I eat a Mediterranean diet, I always lose weight. When I give in to convenience foods and rush through my meals, I always gain weight. It's so predictable!" Eve said.

But Eve is about to turn forty and six months before that date, she started to make some permanent changes in her diet and in her life, embracing the Mediterranean style for good this time. "I decided I had eaten like a teenager for too many years and it was time to grow up and start eating in a way I know works for me and makes me feel and look better," said Eve. Step by step, Eve has incorporated regular exercise, more outdoor time, sit-down family dinners, and organic, unprocessed food into her diet. She eats a lot of fish but very little meat, and her backyard Iowa garden has supplied her family with lots of peppers, tomatoes, eggplant, salad greens, cilantro, tarragon, and apples from her two apple trees. She visits the farmers' market every week all season and uses olive oil instead of butter or other oils in cooking and on salads. And the changes have been dramatic. "When I write a book, I always practice what I preach, but with this book, I can already tell the changes I've made are going to stick. I already feel younger. My skin looks younger. I have much more energy, and during the writing of this book, I lost fifteen pounds. Best of all, I feel great knowing I am instilling healthy habits and yes, just a little food snobbery, in my children. Whenever they take a bite of something new, I urge them 'Taste! Taste! Don't forget to taste!'"

Eve teaches her sons how to cook, how to choose fresh fruits and vegetables, and how to appreciate foods most kids don't normally eat in America. Eve's seven-year-old son, Emmett, recently made a comment that reminded Eve of Melissa's early childhood experiences in the school lunchroom. Emmett said, "Mom, why do you put this stuff in my lunch? Can't I have normal food? None of the other kids have cold salmon. None of the other kids even know what salmon is!" Eve just smiled and answered, "Well then, don't you feel sorry for those other kids? You know, you're the lucky one."

Cranberry Cornmeal Cookies

Makes about 3 dozen

These satisfying cookies have a sparkling crunch from the cornmeal and a tart chewiness from the dried cranberries.

¾ pound unsalted butter, at room temperature
1½ cups sugar
2 eggs
2 teaspoons vanilla extract

3 cups unbleached all-purpose flour
1 cup cornmeal
2 teaspoons baking powder
½ teaspoon salt
2 cups dried cranberries

1. Preheat the oven to 350°F. Put the butter and sugar into a large bowl and cream them together until fluffy using a stand or handheld mixer.

2. Add the eggs one at a time and beat well after each addition. Beat in the vanilla.

3. In a separate large bowl, whisk together the flour, cornmeal, baking powder, and salt. Stir the dry ingredients into the butter mixture, mixing just until combined. Stir in the cranberries.

4. Cover a baking sheet with parchment paper or a Silpat baking mat. Roll the dough into 1-inch balls and flatten them. Place them on the baking sheet about 2 inches apart.

5. Bake until the cookies are golden brown, 8–10 minutes. Watch them and be sure not to overbrown. They should be crispy but not dried out. Cool 10 minutes, then carefully remove the cookies to a wire cooling rack. Serve warm or at room temperature.

Almond Biscotti

Makes about 3 dozen

Biscotti is among the most versatile of cookies. Perfect with morning coffee, afternoon coffee or tea, or after dinner with coffee or a *digestivo*, biscotti isn't too sweet, is pleasingly crunchy, and is shaped perfectly for dipping. Don't be put off by the fact that you have to bake this twice—once for the loaf, once for the slices. This is still easier than dropping two dozen globs of sticky dough one at a time from a spoon. Try it!

2¼ cups unbleached all-purpose flour

1¾ cups sugar

½ teaspoon salt

1 teaspoon baking powder

1½ teaspoons orange zest

3 eggs

3 egg yolks (reserve egg whites for another use)

1 teaspoon almond extract

7 ounces whole almonds with skins

1 tablespoon orange flower water (optional, available in Middle Eastern grocery stores)

1. Preheat the oven to 325°F. In a large mixing bowl, combine the flour, sugar, salt, baking powder, and orange zest. Set aside.

2. In another large mixing bowl, combine the eggs, egg yolks, and almond extract. Mix thoroughly with a fork or whisk. Stir in the almonds and orange flower water, if using.

3. Add the egg mixture to the flour mixture and combine, stirring with a wooden spoon, just until the dough comes together. Don't overmix.

4. On a large baking sheet, form the dough into two loaves, about 4 inches by 10 inches each. Bake for 20 minutes until lightly browned. Let the biscotti loaves cool. When they are just

slightly warm, slice them with a sharp serrated knife into ½-inch slices.

5. Lower the oven temperature to 300°F. Put the slices, cut sides up so they lie flat, back on the baking sheet. Bake for 15 minutes, or until the slices are golden and dry. Serve warm or at room temperature.

Lavender Shortbread

Makes about 3 dozen

This unusual lavender-scented cookie gives shortbread an exotic twist. You can find dried lavender flowers in the bulk herb section of specialty stores and co-op health food stores, or grow it yourself in your herb garden. The scent of lavender is soothing and relaxing. This is a fun recipe to do with kids because it is easy, quick, and you get to use cookie cutters!

½ pound unsalted butter, at room
    temperature
½ cup sugar
2 cups unbleached all-purpose flour,
    plus more for dusting

Pinch of salt
2 tablespoons dried lavender

1. Combine the butter and sugar in a mixing bowl and beat until combined using a stand or handheld mixer. Add the flour and salt, and mix on low speed until the mixture resembles wet sand.

2. Add the lavender and mix just until the dough starts to come together.

3. Turn out the dough onto a flour-dusted pastry board or clean countertop and gather it into a mass. Roll it out so that it is about ¼ inch thick. Cut it out with small cookie cutters.

4. Carefully move the cookies with a metal spatula onto a Silpat- or parchment-covered baking sheet and chill in the refrigerator for 1 hour.

5. Preheat the oven to 275°F. Bake the chilled cookies until they are crisp and dry, 20–25 minutes. Remove from the baking sheet after five minutes and cool on a wire cooling rack.

French Almond Wafers

These delicate cookies use ground almonds instead of flour, so they have a lacy texture and that perfect almond flavor. This is a very simple cookie without any flavoring other than the almonds. You can pipe whipped cream inside the cookies just before serving, but they are good without it, too. Serve them with sherry, champagne, or little glass dishes of fruit salad. They also go well with gelato, of course. (What doesn't?)

4 ounces blanched almonds sugar
¼ pound unsalted butter, at room temperature

1 tablespoon unbleached all-purpose flour
2 tablespoons milk

1. Preheat the oven to 350°F. Grind the almonds in a blender or spice grinder until they are very fine.

2. Put all the ingredients together in a saucepan over low heat. Stir gently until the butter is melted and everything is fully incorporated.

3. Remove from the heat and scoop spoonfuls about 2 inches apart onto a Silpat- or parchment-lined baking sheet. Bake for 5–8 minutes, or until barely golden brown. Turn each wafer over with a metal spatula. Return to the oven and bake an additional 5 minutes, or until well browned.

4. Let the wafers cool for 2 minutes. Then carefully roll each wafer around a form into a tube. You can use ½-inch wooden dowels or any other cylindrical form you can find; or roll them into a cone shape, or just leave them flat.

Socca

French street food, socca is a kind of fried bread made from chickpea flour. It can also be cooked into a porridge, chilled, sliced, and fried like polenta, but in this recipe, you ladle the batter into a pan and fry it like a pancake. Serve it plain or with salad, olives, and cheese for a light lunch.

1½ cups chickpea flour	1 tablespoon chopped fresh sage
2 cups water	½ teaspoon sea salt
⅔ cup extra-virgin olive oil	Freshly ground black pepper to taste

1. Mix all the ingredients except ⅓ cup of the extra-virgin olive oil together in a large bowl. Cover with plastic wrap or a tea towel and let the batter rest for 1 hour.

2. Heat an 8-inch nonstick sauté pan over medium-high heat. Add 1 tablespoon of the remaining olive oil. When it is hot, ladle in ¼ cup of the batter. Roll it around with the ladle to spread it thinly over the bottom of the pan, as you would do when cooking a crepe. Cook until brown and crispy on the edges, 5–7 minutes.

3. Repeat with the remaining batter, adding a tablespoon (or less) of olive oil before each new addition of batter.

✳ Frozen Desserts

All over Europe, especially in the cities, you can find gelato stands — Italy's answer to ice cream. In the early evening, everybody walking the streets seems to flock to them. There is something lovely about strolling through the Mediterranean at dusk with a scoop of flavorful gelato. You can now buy gelato from vendors in many cities in the United States, too. In the Mediterranean, most women don't make gelato themselves at home, but if you have an ice-cream maker, you can make it pretty easily. You can also make sorbetto, the Italian version of sorbet, which is much lower in fat because it contains no egg yolks, cream, or milk. Sorbetto is a good dessert. In its citrus incarnation, it makes an excellent palate cleanser between courses during a formal dinner.

Chocolate Gelato

Gelato can come in any flavor imaginable, but for chocolate lovers, this is Price's basic, beautiful, smooth, creamy recipe for gelato that will give you everything you desire when you crave chocolate. Serve it with any of the cookies in the previous section and you've got a very special dessert.

3 tablespoons unsweetened cocoa
    powder
½ cup minus 1 tablespoon sugar
2½ cups milk

3 egg yolks (reserve whites for another
    use)
1 teaspoon vanilla extract

1. Combine the cocoa powder and half the sugar in a small bowl. Stir in just enough milk to make a paste.

2. Place the rest of the milk in a saucepan and bring it to a boil. Slowly pour about ¼ cup hot milk into the paste, whisking constantly.

3. Stir the paste back into the boiled milk and continue cooking over low heat. Simmer for 5–7 minutes, stirring constantly, then remove from the heat.

4. Beat together the egg yolks and the remaining sugar until pale. Add just a few tablespoons of the hot milk mixture to the yolks while beating. Then add the yolk mixture to the hot milk mixture, beating constantly.

5. Return the pan to the heat and cook over medium until the temperature reaches 185°F (use a candy thermometer clipped to the side of the saucepan). Remove from the heat.

6. Strain the mixture into a large bowl using a fine-mesh strainer. Stir in the vanilla extract. Cover and chill in the refrigerator for at least 2 hours or overnight.

7. Freeze in your ice-cream machine according to the machine's directions. Store in the freezer.

Coconut Sorbetto

Makes about 3 cups

This sorbet tastes creamy because of the coconut milk but also tangy and exotic because of the lime juice. It is very easy to make and will impress people when they discover you made it yourself. The coconut makes this sorbetto rich, so you need only a small scoop to get your fill.

One 14- or 15-ounce can cream of coconut

Two 13.5-ounce cans coconut milk

¾ cups simple syrup (¾ cup water and ¾ cup sugar boiled together until sugar dissolves)

¾ cup water

2 tablespoons freshly squeezed lime juice

1. Combine all the ingredients in a large mixing bowl and mix well with a hand blender.

2. Strain the mixture through a fine sieve. Cover and chill for at least 2 hours or overnight.

3. Freeze in your ice-cream machine according to the machine's directions. Store in the freezer.

✳ Cakes, Custards, and Creams

Baking doesn't have to be hard, although it can be more important to measure ingredients exactly when baking than when, say, making a pot of soup. Making a cake for your family is a real gift, so try one of these recipes if you have a free afternoon. Exacting measurements also apply to making custards and creams. Popular desserts in the Mediterranean include panna cotta and zabaglione in Italy, crème brûlée in France, flan in Spain, rice pudding and Turkish custard on the Mediterranean's eastern shore, and millet porridge from North Africa.

Crema Catalana

This creamy, rich custard is the Spanish version of crème brûlée. Custard is a popular dessert in Spain. Flavorful and full of protein and calcium, these little dishes of custard topped with a thin brown-sugar crust make the perfect small, elegant dessert.

1½ cups milk

1½ cups cream

Freshly grated zest from 4 oranges

Freshly grated zest from 2 lemons

½ vanilla bean

1 cinnamon stick

½ cup sugar

8 egg yolks (reserve whites for another use)

2 tablespoons unbleached all-purpose flour

6 teaspoons fine granulated sugar for topping

1. Combine the milk, cream, orange and lemon zests, the vanilla bean (scrape the seeds into the milk mixture with a sharp knife first, then drop in the pod), and the cinnamon stick together in a large saucepan. Place over medium heat and warm the mixture until it almost simmers. Don't let it boil. Cook without boiling until the mixture begins to thicken, about 30 minutes.

2. In a bowl, whisk the sugar and egg yolks together. Stir in the flour.

3. While whisking the yolk mixture constantly, very slowly add about ½ cup of the hot milk mixture in a small, steady stream. Keep whisking so the yolks don't cook. Then slowly add the yolk mixture, in the same way, into the pan of hot milk, whisking the milk constantly as you add it. Bring the mixture to a very gentle simmer, whisking steadily, for 3 more minutes, or until the mixture thickens slightly.

4. Strain the custard through a fine-mesh strainer into a glass measuring cup with a spout, then pour the custard into six ceramic ramekins or other small ceramic dishes. Let the custard chill for 2–3 hours, or preferably overnight, until it is set and completely cold.

5. To serve, top each custard with 1 teaspoon of the fine granulated sugar and place under the broiler for 2–3 minutes, or until the sugar caramelizes (or use a cooking torch, if you have one). Watch it carefully so you don't burn the sugar. Serve immediately, as is or topped with chopped seasonal fruit.

Easy Brioche

This is Price's recipe for brioche, a tender, egg-rich (high-protein) bread dough that can be shaped any way you like it. You can make it in a loaf pan, shape it into a round loaf and bake it on a baking sheet, or you can make individual brioche buns, which is a nice way to control serving size. You can bake these on a baking sheet or in muffin tins. This is a flexible dough that you can adapt any way you like. Some people like brioche plain with a little butter, which is good if you want something baked but not too sweet. Or you might make an indentation in the centers and fill the brioche with jam or custard. Some recipes add chocolate or even chopped fresh fruit into the dough. I like brioche plain, warm with a cup of tea. Try this recipe out in its pure form, and once you've got it down, you can start experimenting with what you might add to make your brioche more to your taste. Make the individual brioche rolls small and enjoy just one for a snack or dessert, and you won't have to worry about getting too much fat.

1 pound plus ¹/4 cup unsalted butter

5 eggs

2 tablespoons active dry yeast (or two packets)

6 tablespoons sugar

2 teaspoons salt

2 tablespoons milk

2¹/4 cups high-gluten flour (bread flour)

1. Put all the ingredients in a mixing bowl and mix using a stand or handheld mixer until the sides of the bowl are clean. Refrigerate the dough overnight.

2. Preheat the oven to 350°F. Divide the chilled dough into 24 pieces. Roll each piece into a ball.

3. Place the dough on a lightly greased baking sheet or Silpat-lined baking sheet, about 2 inches apart, or put the balls of dough into lightly greased individual muffin tins.

4. Bake until the rolls are light golden brown, 18–20 minutes. Cool on a wire cooling rack and store covered for up to 2 days.

Olive Oil and Lemon–Scented Semolina Cake

Serves 12

This cake may sound unusual to you, but it isn't at all unusual to women living in the Mediterranean. In Italy and particularly in Greece, it is quite common to bake with olive oil instead of butter. Italians also like to use semolina flour—traditional for pasta—in their cakes for a denser, grainier texture. This is a filling, delicious cake that requires little garnishment. A small slice with coffee or tea makes a satisfying afternoon snack. However, if you want to fancy it up for a special occasion, top each slice with a small scoop of sorbetto, such as the Coconut Sorbetto earlier in this chapter, and a little bitter chocolate shaved over the top. I also like to drizzle the plate with chilled Pineapple Syrup (recipe follows).

4 large eggs, at room temperature

3/4 cup sugar

Zest of 1 lemon

2/3 cup extra-virgin olive oil

1 1/4 cups unbleached all-purpose flour

1/4 cup semolina flour

1 tablespoon baking powder

1/2 teaspoon salt

Optional garnishes: Pineapple Syrup (recipe follows), Coconut Sorbetto (page 297), bittersweet chocolate shaved with a vegetable peeler, mint sprigs

1. Preheat the oven to 325°F. Put the eggs into a large bowl and beat them with a stand or handheld mixer until combined. Switch to the whip attachment and whip for 1 minute.

2. Slowly add the sugar and whip until the entire mixture is very pale and frothy. Mix in the lemon zest.

3. In a separate bowl, mix together the olive oil, flours, baking powder, and salt. Add the sugar mixture in two batches to the flour mixture, mixing just until combined. Do not overmix.

4. Grease a ring mold or bundt-type pan. Pour the batter into the pan. Bake until lightly browned, 25–35 minutes. A skewer should come out moist.

5. Cool on a wire rack. Serve warm or at room temperature. To assemble the dessert for more formal occasions, drizzle chilled pineapple syrup on individual dessert plates. Top with a slice of warm cake. Place a small scoop of coconut (or other flavor) sorbetto on top of each cake slice, then top that with a few shavings of bittersweet chocolate. Garnish with a sprig of mint.

Pineapple Syrup

Makes about 1 cup

This syrup enriches any cake, or try it drizzled over coconut sorbetto for a refreshingly tropical dessert. Keep it in a glass jar in the refrigerator for up to two weeks.

¾ of a large pineapple, skinned, cored, and cut into 1-inch-thick slices
¾ cup simple syrup (¾ cup water and ¾ cup sugar boiled together until sugar dissolves)
½ vanilla bean, split in half
2 tablespoons golden rum, plus more if needed
2 tablespoons freshly squeezed lemon juice, plus more if needed

1. Put the pineapple into a large saucepan. Add the simple syrup. Scrape the seeds from the vanilla bean into the pot, then add the vanilla bean, too. Cook over medium-low heat until the fruit is tender and cooked through.

2. Process the mixture in a food processor or use an immersion blender in the saucepan. Strain the syrup into a bowl through a fine sieve.

3. Stir in the rum and lemon juice. Adjust to taste. Chill at least 2 hours or overnight.

Panna Cotta

This smooth, creamy panna cotta is very basic. Unlike a custard, it does not contain eggs and you don't have to bake it. It gets its thick, tangy creaminess from yogurt, and this is a delicious way to eat yogurt. Panna cotta is easily dressed up with fresh herbs such as lemon verbena, mint, or lavender, a thin, crunchy cookie, and whatever fresh fruit is in season.

½ cup whole-milk yogurt plus 1½ cups yogurt (you can use sheep's, goat's, or cow's milk yogurt)

2 tablespoons and 2 teaspoons plus ½ cup heavy cream or milk
1½ teaspoons powdered gelatin
½ cup sugar

1. Lightly oil five 4-ounce ramekins or molds with a flavorless oil such as canola.

2. Combine ½ cup yogurt and the 2 tablespoons and 2 teaspoons heavy cream or milk in a medium stainless steel bowl. Whisk to combine. Sprinkle the gelatin over the mixture and set it aside to expand and begin to gel.

3. Meanwhile, heat the remaining ½ cup heavy cream or milk and the sugar in a saucepan over medium heat. Bring to a boil to dissolve the sugar. Stir this mixture into the mixture with the gelatin.

4. Set a saucepan of water over medium-high heat and bring to a boil. Place the bowl of yogurt–cream–gelatin mixture over the boiling water and stir until the gelatin is completely dissolved. This could take 15 minutes.

5. Remove the bowl from the heat and whisk in the remaining 1½ cups yogurt. Mix until thoroughly combined.

6. Strain the mixture through a fine-mesh sieve or cheesecloth and pour it into the oiled ramekins or molds. Put them on a tray, cover them lightly with plastic wrap, and set them in the refrigerator to chill for at least 2 hours or overnight. To serve, run a small paring knife around the edge of each mold and turn it out gently onto a dessert plate. Garnish with fresh herbs, fresh fruit, pineapple syrup, or just enjoy in its pure form.

If you love coffee with your dessert, you can easily fit this warming and stimulating beverage into a Mediterranean lifestyle. Different countries have different coffee traditions. Coffee is a passion in the Mediterranean. Coffee with milk accompanies breakfast, while espresso makes a good afternoon pick-me-up as well as an after-dinner drink. And coffee is good for you! A recent study listed coffee as the number-one source of antioxidants in the American diet. Coffee's concentrated antioxidants may protect against certain cancers and other diseases of aging. Coffee also lowers your risk of type 2 diabetes, increases cognitive abilities, and is a proven mood and performance booster. No wonder we love it so much!

In the eastern Mediterranean, coffee is often prepared with sugar and spices such as cardamom, and it is very strong, served in small demitasse cups. Turkish coffee is a perfect example. Our friend Lydia comes from Lebanon. Her Lebanese coffee recipe is provided here. Lydia says that in Lebanon, the hostess typically adds sugar according to individual guest preferences. Each cup of coffee is usually served with a glass of water on a serving tray, frequently along with a tiny piece of chocolate or other sweets. Coffee is always served to visitors following lunch. "Lebanese women don't consider a visit complete without coffee," counsels Lydia.

• •

LYDIA'S LEBANON

In Lebanon, says our friend Lydia, who now lives in the United States, the diet is fresh and diverse. "Because we live on the Mediterranean Sea, Lebanon enjoys a large variety of fish and shellfish . . . and even sea turtles. Our diet is rich in wheat such as bulgur, vegetables of many choices, rice, and beans. Fruits are essential to our diet and are served instead of desserts after the main meals." Spices also play a big part in Lebanese cuisine, says Lydia. "Allspice, black pepper, and cinnamon are always used in our cooking, and so is garlic, in almost every dish. And onions!" Red meat and chicken are featured in some meals. Food is incredibly important to the people of Lebanon.

"Cooking is time-consuming, as Lebanese people like to celebrate with fancy food and are first-class gourmets. They work it off in a party of belly dancing, which is very popular in Lebanon," Lydia says with a laugh. Almost every night people go out to dance."

• •

Lydia's Lebanese Coffee

Lydia tells us this recipe originated in Turkey many centuries ago. The Arabic name of the coffee pot traditionally used to make this coffee is Rakwa, and it comes in different sizes. You can find these coffee pots in Middle Eastern stores, and more often than not, in good general-purpose kitchen stores, too.

2 demitasse-sized cups of water
½ teaspoon sugar (optional)

Pinch of cardamom (optional)
2 teaspoons coffee, very finely ground

1. In a small saucepan over high heat, boil the water with the optional sugar.

2. Add the cardamom, if using, and coffee. Boil several more times, lifting the saucepan up every time the coffee reaches the boiling point to lower the heat. Pour into demitasse cups and serve hot or warm.

Now wasn't that sweet? Remember that dessert is one of the most pleasurable parts of a celebratory meal, but it simply isn't a regular part of Mediterranean meals on a daily basis. Many women do have a very small sweet in the afternoon with coffee, but that would be the only sweet of the day. If you reserve sweets for special occasions, they really do become something very special.

16

Long Life!

Que será, será...
Whatever will be, will be . . .

For centuries, women have dreamed of a fountain of youth, a key to eternal life, and the best ways to live a long and healthy existence. All we need do is look to the Mediterranean, where women often live beyond a hundred years, comfortable, cared for, and healthy.

The Mediterranean lifestyle holds the secret. It is the fountain of youth. Caring for our body, mind, and spirit with good food, exercise, fresh air, strong families, and enduring friendships will nurture us into old age. We will be able to remain beautiful, healthy, connected to society, and well respected in the tradition of the Mediterranean, where everyone presumes that "older" automatically means "wiser," and the oldest family members are cherished as active, vibrant components of family life.

You don't have to quote statistics to a Mediterranean woman

about life spans and how many extra years may grace a Mediterranean woman's life because of the way she eats, how she moves, how she thinks about life—she sees it around her in the lovely character of the old faces and agility of the old hands of women, still cooking, still laughing, still loving through generations of family, *living* a hundred years and beyond!

Sometimes, when I think about life in the United States, I think it seems very far away from life in the Mediterranean. But at other times, I think we almost have it right, as I wander through the tea garden or pick flowers for the tables or wave hello to my neighbors or greet the regular customers that travel from all around to come to Primo for dinner, where they know they will be nurtured with good food that is prepared with love. I'm living the Mediterranean life, right here in coastal Maine, and you can live it, too, no matter where you live, even if you are miles from the sea.

As the American writer Charlotte Cushman once wrote, "To try to be better is to be better." Taking these tiny, pleasurable steps toward a better life can make big differences in the way we look, feel, and embrace life. What better source for advice than the ancient wisdom of the Mediterranean? Everything you do to adjust your life to a healthier, more natural way of living can add years to your life and make you feel better, healthier, more energetic, right now.

It could well be that the best years of your life are yet to come. Let's quickly review some of the ways in which the Mediterranean way of life can help you to live longer and better. This is advice, pure and simple, from me to you, encompassing everything in this book that I think is truly crucial for embracing the Mediterranean diet, lifestyle, and spirit:

• A thermos of hot homemade soup is better than a Twinkie, anytime, anywhere.

- You can be different from many other people with their bad food habits and convenience store mentality. You can be yourself, however and whoever you are.

- The Mediterranean is a land of individualism. Be who *you* want to be, not who someone tells you to be. You don't have to pretend to be French or Italian or Greek or anything other than who you are right here, right now.

- You can change if you decide to change. Breaking bad habits is not the same as changing your personality.

- To know who you are and who you want to be, slow down. Stop. Look around you. Breathe. Pay attention. Don't miss your life!

- Take a hard look at your own relationship with food. How is it negative? It's okay to *love* food, really love it. Food should never make you feel guilty.

- Garlic can make your life better.

- When you don't know what to eat, choose something that grows from the earth.

- If you always have a jar of pepperonata and a loaf of good bread in the house, you will always know what to eat.

- Yogurt can make your life better.

- Eat a little bit of a lot of things rather than a lot of just a few things. Variety really is the spice of life.

- Eat according to what's in season. Learn what's in season and when.

- Eat what is grown nearby rather than what has been shipped from hundreds or thousands of miles away. Always choose the fresh, local, native foods first.

- Shop at farmers' markets, produce stands, and food co-ops.

- Meet the people who produce the food you eat. Get to know them. Talk to them.

- If you want to know something in life, ask.

- Don't buy food wrapped in plastic and Styrofoam. You should be able to pick it up, look at it, smell it, and *interact* with it before you shell out your hard-earned cash for it.

- Protein doesn't just come from meat. Grains, beans, peas, nuts, yogurt, and cheese are full of it. Eat some of these foods every day.

- A good soup, a good salad, and a little bread make a very good meal.

- Flavor is more important than quantity.

- Quality is more important than quantity.

- Vegetables can be the main course. Make them a big part of your meals.

- Vegetables taste great when you grill them.

- Vegetables are the most interesting food items out there. You have an entire universe of vegetables to choose from, and every single one has its charms.

- Whole grains are the staff of life and are by no stretch of the imagination "evil," despite what you might have heard.

- Fruit *is* dessert.

- A little fat is good for you.

- Of all the types of fat in the world, extra-virgin olive oil is the very best one.

- The fats that come in almonds and walnuts win second prize.

- No matter where you live, you can grow some sort of garden if you want to.

- If you don't want to grow a garden, you don't have to. Plenty of other people will do it for you, and you can support them by buying what they grow.

- Nurturing a garden can make you a better person.

- The vegetables you grow yourself taste better than the vegetables in the grocery store.

- Growing herbs is a spiritual pursuit.

- Eggs can be the main course.

- Organic eggs taste better than factory-farmed eggs.

- Little tastes can add up to an entire meal without any "main course" at all.

- Anchovies must not be feared. They are very small. And very tasty. Use them as seasoning.

- Sometimes, even flowers make good food.

- Sheep's and goat's milk make for excellent cheeses and superior yogurts.

- You don't have to eat a lot of meat to really enjoy meat.

- You don't have to eat meat every day.

- Eating meat about once or twice a week does not make you a vegetarian, but it does make you healthier.

- If you can eat a chicken, you can eat a duck. If you can eat a duck, you can eat a rabbit.

Long Life!
~ 315 ~

- Just because you haven't tried something does not mean you don't like it!

- Not having tried something before is a very good reason to try it now.

- Fish is a gift from the sea.

- There are plenty of fish in the sea besides salmon.

- There is more than one kind of salmon.

- Eating with your family is better than eating alone.

- Feeding your family and friends is an act of love.

- Your food tastes better if you cook it with care, attention, and love.

- Even if they irritate you sometimes, your family is a gift.

- Friends can be just like family.

- Let others help you cook. No kitchen is too small for willing helpers.

- Laughing is good for your digestion.

- On certain days, you might really need to eat meat and potatoes. On other days, you might need little but fresh vegetables and fruits.

- Prepare your body and mind for dinner by relaxing with an *aperitivo* before sitting down to eat.

- Always sit down to eat.

- The television is not a worthy dinner companion.

- Drink a little wine with your dinner, but only with your dinner, not before or after.

- Wine can make your food taste better.

- Help your digestion along with a sweet or bitter *digestivo* after dinner.

- You can end your meal with a good salad.

- You can have a nice piece of cheese for dessert.

- Sometimes a snack is enough.

- You can have your dessert and eat it, too. But you really don't need more than a few bites.

- Even when you think you need more than a few bites of dessert, you really don't. Even so, dessert is a very nice invention.

- You are part of Nature, lest you forget. Look around and see.

- Go outside and breathe.

- Walk more.

- Whatever it is—the good, the bad—tell your friends about it.

- Listen.

- Call your family.

- Play with your kids. They want you more than "stuff."

- Slow down.

- Wake up.

- Look.

- Let go.

- Listen to your body.

- Let yourself be healthy.

- Let yourself be happy.

- Let yourself love.

- Let yourself be passionate.

- Let yourself be slim.

- Take pleasure.

- Taste.

- Live like you mean it.

Omega

Omega is the last letter in the Greek alphabet, the end of a journey, a finishing. But in a way, omega is also a return to the beginning. While we may be at the end of this book's story, it is just a beginning for the new life you can embrace today.

I am right here with you, living this life and embracing this love affair with food I've lived ever since my childhood. And I've always stayed slim. But even if this Mediterranean attitude and way of life is new to you, vitality and a slender body are achievable simply by embracing the spirit of the Mediterranean. It's never too late to begin. You can start right now. I hope you will.

The Mediterranean way of life is so full of pleasure and passion that I would hate for you to miss out on even one more day of this simple, beautiful, flavorful living. Whether you are at a healthy weight right now and are looking for a way to maintain it, or you are looking for a good, permanent way to lose extra weight, the Mediterranean is an ancient source with an enduring secret: *Mediterranean women stay slim, too.* And so can you. Be sexy, fit, and fabulous. Live long, and enjoy life.

Index